ALIVE and WELL

One Doctor's Experience

with Nutrition in the

Treatment of

Cancer Patients

by
Philip E. Binzel, M.D.

American Media

This book is dedicated to my wife Betty who stood by me
through all of the trouble she wouldn't have had in the
first place if she hadn't married me.

Second printing: April, 1996
First printing: October, 1994

Library of Congress Catalog Card Number: 94-079593

ISBN 9780912986173

ACKNOWLEDGMENTS

I am grateful to my six children for their support and generous help in so many ways: Mary Anne and Kathy for giving their time to take care of duties at home so that my wife Betty could be with me during my travels to interviews, hearings, and meetings; Nancy for her outstanding research paper "Nutritional Therapy" which was printed as a booklet for private distribution by my brother-in-law, Philip S. May, Jr.; Bill for his invaluable legal advice during a very serious time; Rick for giving me a computer and teaching me how to use it and for doing the statistical analysis; and my son Ed for being my number one fan.

And my deepest gratitude to the following:

Dr. Ernst Krebs, Jr., who with great patience, taught me everything I know about nutrition.

G. Edward Griffin: Without his urging this book would never have been started and without his encouragement would probably never have been finished.

TABLE OF CONTENTS

Dedication 4

Acknowledgments.................................... 5

Preface 9

Introduction.. 10

Photographs.. 58

Index 141

Chapters

1. Case Dismissed 13

2. The Nutrition Connection 19

3. New Doc on the Block..................................... 27

4. Preparing for Battle............................. 33

5. The Battle Begins 39

6. Laetrile and Cyanide 47

7. Debunking the Debunkers............................... 51

8. The Joey Hofbauer Story................................. 67

9. The Media 77

10. Re-Enter the State Medical Board.................... 85

11. The Total Nutritional Program 97

12. Boring Statistics and Exciting Cases 107

13. The Quality of Life............................. 127

14. Treat the Cause, Not the Symptom !...................... 133

Lives of great men all remind us
That we can make our lives sublime
And departing leave behind us
Footprints in the sands of time.
Footprints that perhaps another
Sailing o're life's solemn main
A forlorn and shipwrecked brother
Seeing shall take heart again.

From *The Psalm of Life* by Longfellow

PREFACE

First of all, please understand that all that follows is absolutely and completely the fault of Mr. G. Edward Griffin.

Those of us who have fought for so long to preserve the God-given rights guaranteed us by our Constitution have, for the most part, fought a losing battle. Big Government, with its hoards of bureaucrats, has beaten the "little man" into submission. He must comply with all of its regulations of his business and his life, or else! Usually, if he fights Big Government, he loses.

In my attempts to use nutritional therapy, which includes the use of Laetrile, in the treatment of cancer, I have often been confronted by the Food and Drug Administration and by the State Medical Board. I have fought and, through the grace of God, I have won. For several years Ed Griffin has been after me to write a book. As he put it, "We have won some victories and the people should know about them." So, this book is being written to tell about these victories (and to get Ed off of my back). If you don't like the book or any parts of the book, don't blame me. Blame Ed Griffin. He made me do it!

The facts in this book are true. The names are real (except where I say they are not). The dates may not be completely accurate, but they are as close as I can remember.

INTRODUCTION

You are about to discover that the author of this book is no ordinary doctor. He is one of those rare birds that is able to leave the flock and fly alone. He has rejected the comforts and rewards of conformity and has chosen instead the hard path of integrity. In order to practice medicine as his conscience dictates, he has literally had to take on the entire medical Establishment. And, as you will see, it has been an uneven battle. The Establishment hasn't had a chance.

Dr. Binzel's motive for writing this book is almost unbelievable in today's world: he simply wants to share his knowledge so that lives can be saved. At the end of a long and successful career, he is not seeking to attract patients. In fact, he is now officially retired. He does consult with patients and their doctors from time to time, but usually at no charge. His present role is that of pioneer and teacher.

Binzel comes from the small town of Washington Court House, Ohio. He is a classical small-town doctor, and that's exactly the way he writes. But do not be deceived. He is at the cutting edge of medical knowledge, and there are few people from the scientific community—regardless of their impressive credentials—who are willing to debate with him a *second* time. His folksy style and

10

genuine humility are refreshing, but he knows his craft exceedingly well.

The title of this book, *Alive and Well,* is appropriate for three reasons. First, there is the happy record of the patients who have received Dr. Binzel's care. Many of them previously had been told by their original physicians that there was no hope for survival, that their cancers were "terminal," and that they had, at best, only a few more months to live. To them, many years later, the phrase *alive and well* has a meaning that only those who have faced death can fully appreciate.

A second significance to the title is the fact that the use of Laetrile in the treatment of cancer is also alive and well—in spite of the fact that it has not been featured in the national news media since the height of its controversy in the late 1970s. Because it has not been on the evening news, many people have assumed that the treatment had been abandoned. As this story demonstrates, however, nothing could be further from the truth.

Finally, there is the fact that Dr. Binzel, himself, is alive and well in the sense that he has survived an incredible barrage of attacks from the medical Establishment. That, in fact, is an important part of this story. Until one understands the political power wielded by drug-oriented medicine and how that power is used against any physician who favors nutritional therapy, it is impossible to understand why nutritional therapy is not widely available to the general public.

Dr. Binzel does not use the word "cured" in describing the condition of his patients who have returned to normal life after treatment. That is more a question of semantics than substance. It is true that, once a person has developed full-blown clinical cancer—even after all their symptoms have vanished—they will have a greater-than-normal tendency to develop cancer again. That, however, assumes they return to their original life styles and eating habits. On the other hand, if they do continue to follow the dietary regimen described in this book, they will throw off that handicap.

So the question remains—are they *cured*? Who cares what word is used if the patient is *alive and well*? In orthodox medicine, they often speak of cures, but the patients are dead! According to the death certificates, they don't die of cancer, but of heart failure, lung failure, liver failure, or hemorrhage. But what caused these? They are the secondary effects of their *treatments* for cancer. "We got it all," is a common refrain. "I'm happy to report that we cured him of his disease—just before he died." This is not really a joke. It is the reality of orthodox cancer therapy.

What you are about to read is a radical departure from that scenario. Be prepared for a deep breath of fresh air.

G. Edward Griffin

Case Dismissed

Chapter One

It was early December, 1977. My office girl, Ruthie Coe, called me on my intercom to tell me that I had a phone call from a Mr. Robert Bradford in California. She wanted to know if I wanted to take the call now or to call him back. I had known Bob Bradford for about three years. He was the head of an organization known as The Committee for Freedom of Choice in Cancer Therapy. I had done several seminars on nutrition with him. I told Ruthie that I would take the call now.

Bob told me that the Food and Drug Administration (The FDA) had filed suit in Federal Court to prohibit the importation of Laetrile into this country because it was toxic. He said that he had found an eminent toxicologist, Dr. Bruce Halstead, who was willing to testify against the FDA, but he also needed a practicing physician who had used Laetrile and wanted to know if I would testify. I told him I would. Bob told me that the hearing would be in Oklahoma City in the court of Judge Luther Bohanon in about ten or twelve days.

I called our local travel agency and asked them to get airplane reservations for my wife, Betty, and me. I knew without talking to her that Betty would not want to miss out on the fun! The girl from the travel agency called me back in a few minutes. She said that she had no problem getting us a flight into Oklahoma City, but a *big* problem getting us out of Oklahoma City. The hearing was, I believe, to be on a Thursday. I wanted to arrive sometime on Wednesday afternoon. Not knowing how long the hearing would take on Thursday, I thought that if we planned to leave on Friday morning, that would work out well. The problem with the airlines was that the University of Oklahoma and all the colleges around the area were starting their Christmas vacation on that Friday. There were no seats available on any airline going in our direction until the following Monday. The last plane leaving Oklahoma City going in our direction that had any space was a three o'clock flight on Thursday afternoon. 1 took those reservations.

Betty and I flew out of Columbus, Ohio to St. Louis. There we changed to a flight to Oklahoma City. On our flight to Oklahoma City (coach, of course), I noticed that there were only three men flying first class. At that time, I don't think the word "clone" had been invented. If it had, these three men certainly could have been described as clones of each other. They were all about the same height, weight, hair color, and all had the same haircut. They all had the same sallow complexion, wore the same black suits and maroon ties, and they all carried the same type of briefcase.

Early the next morning Bob Bradford, Dr. Halstead, Betty and I met with the attorney, Mr. Ken Coe, (no relation to my office girl, Ruthie Coe). I told Mr. Coe of our predicament with our airline schedule. He assured me that he would discuss this with the Judge and do whatever he could to help.

While we were sitting there, Mr. Coe received a phone call. It seems that there had been a young girl in New York

CASE DISMISSED

who, some months before, had gotten hold of a bottle of Laetrile pills belonging to her father and had taken an unknown quantity of these. She was taken to a hospital and a number of blood tests were done over the next two days. The girl exhibited no symptoms, but, for whatever reason, on the third day the doctors decided to give her the antidote to cyanide. The girl died the following day.

From what I know, the FDA had contacted the girl's mother and wanted her to testify about the toxicity of Laetrile. She had refused but said, instead, that she would testify against the FDA. She had flown out of New York early that Thursday morning and was due to arrive in Oklahoma City about nine o'clock. It was she who was calling to let us know that about two or three hundred miles out of New York someone on the plane had a heart attack. The plane turned around and went back to New York. She was not going to be able to get to Oklahoma City. Mr. Coe said, "We'll go with what we've got."

We arrived in the court room shortly before nine o'clock. The first thing that I noticed were the three "clones" I had seen on the airplane the day before. They were the FDA attorneys. Why were there three of them? A friend of mine explained that to me sometime later. He said that, in case they lose, each attorney always puts the blame on the other two! The thing that bothered me the most was that Betty and I had to pay our own air fare, and we flew coach. My taxes were paying their air fare, and they flew first class.

Judge Bohanon entered the court room. Mr. Coe, as promised, immediately asked for and received permission to approach the bench. He explained to the Judge the problem that Betty and I had with airline reservations. Judge Bohanon very kindly agreed to change the usual procedure and to allow the defense to present its case first.

I testified first. Responding to Mr. Coe's questions, I stated that I had used Laetrile both by mouth and by intravenous injection on several hundred patients, and that I had not experienced any toxic reaction in any of those patients. On cross-examination the FDA attorney asked me if I was familiar with the term "agmpxyztpwrquos" (or something like that). I said, "No." He then asked if I was familiar with the term "mvchrtonlxty" (or something like that). Again, I said, "No." I was then dismissed from the witness stand. To this day, I do not know the meaning of the two terms. The FDA attorney never gave the definitions. I had never heard the terms before and have never heard them since. I am not sure that they didn't just make up two terms to see if I would bite.

Dr. Halstead then took the stand. He carried with him a book which he put in his lap. Under direct questioning from Mr. Coe, Dr. Halstead explained how all substances known to man can be toxic. He showed that while some oxygen is necessary to maintain life, too much oxygen can be fatal. He went through the same procedure with water, salt, and other substances. He then showed that aspirin, sugar and salt were, milligram-for-milligram, more toxic than Laetrile. He further pointed out that chemotherapeutic agents which are commonly used in the treatment of cancer are, milligram-for-milligram, hundreds of times more toxic than Laetrile.

On cross-examination, the FDA attorney asked Dr. Halstead to give the toxicity figure for some substance (I don't remember what the substance was). Dr. Halstead said, pointing to the book in his lap but never opening it, "On page 311, Table 2, in this book you will find that the toxicity of that substance is ...." (whatever it was). The FDA attorney then named another substance and asked for its toxicity figure. Dr. Halstead answered, "On page 419,

CASE DISMISSED

Table 3 shows it to be   (whatever it was). The attorney tried a third time. Again, Dr. Halstead came up with the page number, table number and toxicity.

The three FDA attorneys stared at each other for a minute, then one of them said, "How do you know all of this?" Dr. Halstead calmly replied, "Because I wrote the book." "Impossible!" yelled the attorney. Without saying a word, Dr. Halstead took the book from his lap and handed it to Judge Bohanon. The Judge opened the book to its first page and read the following, "Textbook of Toxicology, written by Dr. Bruce Halstead, as commissioned by the Food and Drug Administration of the United States." The Judge said to the FDA attorneys, "You fellows should have known that. You didn't do your homework very well." The FDA attorneys had enough of Dr. Halstead. They dismissed him from the stand.

When Mr. Coe informed Judge Bohanon that the defense had concluded its testimony, the Judge turned to the FDA attorneys and said, "The court is now prepared to hear your witnesses and view your evidence." One FDA attorney replied, "Your Honor, we don't have any." The rest of the dialogue went like this:

Judge: "You are telling me that you have filed suit in this court that Laetrile is toxic, and you don't have a single witness or a shred of evidence to support such a suit?"

Attorney: "That is correct, Your Honor."

Judge: "Then why have you filed such a suit?"

Attorney: "Because, Your Honor, Laetrile may be dangerous."

Judge: "Dangerous to whom?"

Attorney: "Dangerous to the Federal Government, Your Honor."

Judge: "How could Laetrile possibly be dangerous to the Federal Government?"

17

Attorney: "Because, Your Honor, the Government may lose control."

With this the Judge, now obviously angered, slammed down his gavel and said, "Case dismissed!"

As Mr. Coe, Dr. Halstead, Bob Bradford, Betty and I left the court house, we saw a six-foot by four-foot poster on the wall in the lobby. It read in large letters, "BEWARE OF LAETRILE! IT IS TOXIC!" At the bottom, in small print, was the statement, "Must be posted in all Government buildings by order of the Food and Drug Administration of the United States."

Is it possible that the FDA was lying to the people?

The Nutrition Connection

Chapter Two

So, how did a Family Physician from a small town in Ohio ever get involved in a conflict with the FDA in the first place? If you read the *Preface*, you already know the answer. It was the fault of Mr. G. Edward Griffin.

In 1973 I was in the family practice of medicine in Washington Court House, Ohio. I had graduated from St. Louis University School of Medicine in 1953. I did one year of internship and one year of Family Practice residency at Christ Hospital in Cincinnati. In 1955 I began my private practice as a Family Physician in Washington Court House. I was very content with what I was doing until the day a friend of mine, Mr. Charles Pensyl, invited me and a number of others to his camera shop to see a new film that he had just gotten. The title of the film was *World Without Cancer.*

World Without Cancer ran about fifty minutes. It was about a substance called Laetrile and what this substance could do to help people who had cancer. I took a very dim view of this movie because I felt that it made many statements for which there was no supporting medical evidence. The film was produced and narrated by G. Edward Griffin.

ALIVE AND WELL

This caused an immediate problem. As a long time member of the John Birch Society, I had read almost everything that Ed Griffin had written. I had read his book, *The Fearful Master, A Second Look at the United Nations.* I had read numerous articles written by him in the magazine *American Opinion.* He had produced some films, *The Grand Design* and *More Deadly Than War.* All of these, I knew, had been researched extremely well.

To compound the problem, I knew Ed personally. From 1968 through 1972, I served as the doctor for the John Birch Society Youth Camps in Michigan and Indiana. Betty was my assistant. In the first camp that we did, Ed Griffin was the closing speaker. He was to speak on Friday night. He came into camp on Thursday. The staff of the camp was housed in one building. It was the custom of the staff to get together after "lights out" for the campers to discuss the various "opportunities" that had presented themselves that day. (Please note that there was no such thing as a "problem." These were "opportunities.") Ed Griffin attended both the Friday night and Saturday night sessions. I got to know him very well and was impressed with his depth of knowledge on a wide range of subjects.

So, you can see my problem. I didn't think the film *World Without Cancer* was medically accurate, but it was produced and narrated by a man for whom I had the highest respect. I had the feeling he knew something that I didn't know. I felt he would not have produced the film if there was not a great deal more behind this than he was able to show in a fifty-minute film. For three months I vacillated, being sure one minute he was wrong and suspecting the next minute that he just might be right.

Finally, I decided that this mental turmoil had to be resolved. I had a good friend, Steve Michaelis, who was a pharmacist. I called Steve to see what he knew about this

THE NUTRITION CONNECTION

"Laetrile." He was far ahead of me. He told me he had done an in-depth study of Laetrile some months earlier and was convinced that it had merit. He suggested that I contact a group known as The Committee for Freedom of Choice in California. I did. I told the young lady who answered the phone about my doubts about this whole thing, but, if there was information available, I would study it with an open mind.

Within a week, I received a package of material about six inches thick from The Committee for Freedom of Choice. It contained reprints of articles published by Dr. Ernst Krebs, Jr., Dr. Dean Burk of this country, Dr. Hans Nieper of Germany, Dr. Emesto Contreras of Mexico, Dr. Manuel Navarro of the Philippines, Dr. Shigeaki Sakai of Japan and others. Most of these articles had been published in foreign medical journals and had been translated and reprinted. Some of these articles dated back to the early 1950's. It took me eight months to go through and fully understand the significance of what these men had done.

From the time that cancer was first diagnosed (some three hundred to five hundred years ago) to the present, most members of the medical profession have treated this disease using the theory that the tumor is the disease. This theory said that, if you can remove the tumor or destroy the tumor, you will cure the disease. Drs. Krebs, Burk, Nieper, and others said in essence, "*Wrong!*" These men had seen thousands of cancer patients die. They realized that ninety-five percent of these patients had their tumors treated with surgery, and/or radiation, and/or chemotherapy. It was obvious to them that, if removing the tumor or destroying the tumor cured the disease, ninety-five percent of these people would be alive and well. It was, therefore, equally obvious to them that removing the tumor or destroying the tumor did not cure the disease. This meant, of course, that the tumor was not the *cause* of the disease but was merely a *symptom* of the disease.

Let me compare this with appendicitis. The patient with appendicitis complains of pain. The pain is a symptom of this disease. I can give that patient enough morphine or Demerol to stop the pain. Do I then say to the patient, "Your pain is gone. You're cured!" No! I know that the pain will come back, because I have done nothing to correct the condition within the body that is causing the pain. I have to remove the infected appendix in order to treat the cause. These researchers used this same line of reasoning—they said, if you just remove the tumor and don't treat the condition within the body that allowed the tumor to develop in the first place, the tumor will come back. Of course, they are right! The tumor almost always comes back.

These men dug deeper. While each was working independently, they were all happy to share any of their findings with anyone who would listen. One would find something and send it to the others. One would add something to that and send it on. The result of all of this work was that these men found that the body does have a normal defense against cancer, and they were able to describe how that defense mechanism functioned.

They found that the cancer cell is coated with a protein lining, and that it was this protein lining (or covering) that prevented the body's normal defenses from getting to the cancer cell. They found that, if you could dissolve the protein lining from around the cancer cell, the body's normal defenses, the leukocytes (white blood cells), would destroy the cancer cell. They found that the dissolving of the protein lining (or covering) from around the cancer cell was done very nicely within the body by two enzymes: trypsin and chymotrypsin. These enzymes are secreted by the pancreas. Thus, they said that the enzymes trypsin and chymotrypsin formed the body's first line of defense against cancer.

What's an enzyme? I just knew you were going to ask! An enzyme is a catalyst. What's a catalyst? Back in your high school chemistry you were taught the definition of a catalyst. I'm sure that none of you have forgotten that definition. Just in case that definition has (only momentarily, of course) escaped your memory, it is as follows: A catalyst is a substance which causes a chemical reaction to take place without, itself, becoming a part of that chemical reaction. See, I knew you would remember! There are numerous enzymes within the body that are responsible for the hundreds of chemical reactions which must take place in order to keep the body functioning normally. You have now completed Physiology 101.

In addition to finding that trypsin and chymotrypsin formed the body's first line of defense against cancer, Dr. Krebs *et al.* found that the body has a second line of defense against this disease. This second line of defense is formed by a group of substances known as nitrilosides. The cancer cell has an enzyme, beta-glucosidase, which, when it comes in contact with nitrilosides, converts those nitrilosides into two molecules of glucose, one molecule of benzaldehyde and one molecule of hydrogen cyanide. Originally, it was thought that only the hydrogen cyanide was toxic to the cancer cell. Recent evidence has shown that, while the hydrogen cyanide may exert some toxic effect, it is the benzaldehyde that is extremely toxic to the cancer cell.

What is so significant about this is that this is a target-specific reaction. Within the body, the cancer cell and *only* the cancer cell contains the enzyme beta-glucosidase. Thus, the benzaldehyde and the hydrogen cyanide can be formed in the presence of the cancer cell, and *only* the cancer cell. Thus, they are toxic to the cancer cell and only the cancer cell. The normal cell contains the enzyme, rhodanese, which converts the nitrilosides into food.

These researchers found that all of us probably have cancer many times in our lives. If our defense mechanisms are functioning normally, the body kills off the cancer cells, and we're never even aware that it happened. If, however, there is a breakdown in that defense mechanism when the cancer cells appear, there is nothing to prevent the growth of those cancer cells and soon there is a tumor.

What causes a breakdown in that defense mechanism? Suppose you have an individual who is eating large quantities of animal protein. It takes large amounts of the enzymes trypsin and chymotrypsin to digest animal protein. It is possible that this individual is using up all, or almost all, of his trypsin and chymotrypsin for digestive purposes. There is nothing left over for the rest of the body. Thus, this individual has lost his first line of defense against cancer.

Suppose this individual has little or no nitrilosides in his diet. This is quite possible. Millet, which is very high in nitrilosides, used to be the staple grain. We went from millet to wheat, which contains no nitrilosides. Our cattle used to graze and eat large quantities of grasses, which are high in nitrilosides. Now we grain-feed our cattle. There are no nitrilosides in the grain.

So, you now have an individual who, because of his high intake of animal protein, has lost his first line of defense against cancer and who, because of his low intake of nitrilosides, has no second line of defense against cancer. Should cancer cells appear at this time, there is nothing to prevent their growth. The results? Tumor!

THE NUTRITION CONNECTION

As Krebs *et al.* then pointed out, you can remove the tumor, but, if you do not correct the defects in that individual's defense mechanisms, that tumor will come back.

This means that you must markedly reduce the intake of animal protein in these people and replace it with vegetable protein. Vegetable protein requires nothing in the way of the enzymes trypsin and chymotrypsin for digestion. Thus, you can free these enzymes from being used up for digestive purposes, put them back into the body and re-establish the body's first line of defense against cancer.

It means that you must also restore the body's second line of defense against cancer by establishing an adequate level of nitrilosides in these individuals. While there are some 1,500 foods that contain nitrilosides, the researchers found that the most rapid way to build up the nitriloside level was by the use of Laetrile. They did not proclaim Laetrile as a "miracle drug" or a "cancer cure" but merely described it as a concentrated form of nitrilosides, which was able to rapidly raise the nitriloside level and to re-establish the body's second line of defense against cancer.

Perhaps the thing that impressed me most in this large volume of material that I was trying to assimilate, was that all of these researchers stressed the point that cancer was a multiple-variable disease. One of the problems with those of us in the medical profession is that we are used to looking at chronic metabolic diseases (diseases which start within the body, such as diabetes, scurvy, pernicious anemia, pellagra, and cancer) as single-variable diseases. For example, in diabetes, the single-variable deficiency is insulin. In scurvy, it's Vitamin C, and in pernicious

25

anemia, it's B 12. Cancer is a multiple-variable deficiency disease.

These researchers showed that there can be a number of deficiencies within the cancer patient. This, they said, did not mean that all cancer patients had all of these deficiencies, but that any given cancer patient could have six, or eight or ten of these deficiencies. They found, for example, that zinc was the transportation mechanism for the nitrilosides. They found that you could give Laetrile until it came out of the ears of the patient, but, if that patient did not have a sufficient level of zinc, none of the Laetrile would get into the tissues of the body. They also found that nothing heals within the body without sufficient Vitamin C. They found that manganese, magnesium, selenium, Vitamin B, Vitamin A, etc., all played an important part in maintaining the body's defense mechanisms. The most important thing they stressed was that, unless you correct *all* of these deficiencies, you are not going to help that patient. Thus, they were talking about a total nutritional program. They were talking about a program that consisted of diet, vitamins, minerals, enzymes and Laetrile.

New Doc on the Block

Chapter Three

After having spent those eight months studying all of the material sent to me by The Committee for Freedom of Choice, I still was not completely convinced that this nutritional approach to the treatment of cancer would actually work.

I called my pharmacist friend, Steve Michaelis, and learned that Lawrence P. McDonald, M.D., in Atlanta, Georgia, was actively using this form of treatment. I did not know Larry McDonald at that time, but I knew of him. I knew that he was a member of the National Council of the John Birch Society and was a renowned urologist in Atlanta. (This was, of course, the same Rep. Lawrence P. McDonald, Member of Congress, who was on the KAL Flight 007 when it was shot down.) Steve Michaelis knew him very well. Steve called him to let him know that I would be calling.

When we finally talked, Larry could not have been nicer. We discussed at some length the program that he was using. My final question was, "Does it work?" Larry's reply to me was, "If it didn't work, I wouldn't be using it!"

While Larry certainly gave me a push in the right direction, my final decision did not come until I could answer the question, "If I had cancer, or my wife had cancer, or one of my children had cancer, how would I have this treated?" I realized that my answer was, "I'd go with nutritional therapy." It was at that point that I decided to treat my patients with the same method.

Several weeks before I had reached that decision, a very good friend of mine had asked me if I would be willing to give Laetrile to his sister-in-law. This was a hopeless case. The woman had cancer of the breast. In spite of, or maybe because of (depending on your point of view), all the surgery, radiation and chemotherapy that had been done to this woman, she had developed metastases to the liver, lungs and brain. She had been sent home from a Columbus, Ohio hospital and told that she would die within a week or two. She became my first patient. I wish I could say that she lived happily thereafter. She didn't. But she did live for about four months with a minimal amount of pain and suffering.

Within a week after I started treating this first patient, I began to get calls from cancer patients all around this part of the country asking if I would treat them. To this day, I have no idea how those people knew that I was involved in nutritional therapy. I never asked, and they never said.

Most of my first patients were those who had all of the surgery, radiation and chemotherapy they could tolerate and their tumors were still growing. I did for these patients the best that I knew to do.

My biggest problem at this time was understanding nutrition. In four years of medical school, one year of internship and one year of Family Practice residency, I had not had even one lecture on nutrition. How to use the Laetrile, the vitamins and the enzymes was no problem. How to instruct these people on proper nutrition was a big problem. If you know very little about nutrition yourself, how are you to instruct your patients? Simply giving them a diet sheet and saying, "Eat this, but don't eat that," doesn't work. In my years of working with patients with weight problems, I had learned that you never hand a patient a diet sheet. You must explain to the patient why it is necessary to eat certain things and to avoid other things. Once the patient understands this, you then have the patient's full cooperation.

After a few months of using this nutritional program, I was invited by The Committee for Freedom of Choice in Cancer Therapy (and I have no idea how they knew I was using nutritional therapy) to participate in some seminars on nutrition. It was here that I first met Dr. Ernst Krebs. After listening to him for a few minutes, I realized that this man knew more about nutrition then anyone I had ever met.

To say that I presumed on this man's good nature would be the under-statement of the century. I told him what I was doing and how little I knew about nutrition.

These seminars usually lasted for three days and two nights. Dr. Krebs invited me to his room after the first evening's meeting. I was there until the wee hours of the morning and there again until the wee hours of the following morning learning about nutrition. When I think back on all of the stupid questions that I asked, I cannot understand why Dr. Krebs did not bodily pick me up and throw me out of his room. But, I was beginning to learn nutrition.

The second seminar was only a few weeks after the first. Betty was with me on this trip. We started somewhere in the Cleveland area and then flew to St. Louis to do another. Each night Betty, Dr. Krebs and I would get together in Dr. Krebs' room and my education of nutrition would continue.

These seminars went on for several more months. Through the great patience of Dr. Krebs, I became much more comfortable in trying to explain good nutrition to my patients.

When I started using this nutritional approach, I had no pre-conceived ideas of whether it would or would not work. I went into it with a completely open mind. I had decided to try it for one year. If it worked, fine, I would keep it up. If it didn't work, I wouldn't do it any more.

The first thing that I became aware of was that, within a matter of a few weeks, many of the patients were "feeling better." They had less pain and were eating better. While I was not sure that the treatment had added anything to the quantity of the life of these patients, I was sure that it had added something to the *quality* of their lives.

Some of the most beautiful letters that I have received have come from the relatives of patients who have died. They described how wonderful it was that their mother (or sister or brother or wife) had been free of pain and had been able to die comfortably at home rather than in a hospital.

That was encouraging, so I continued. Toward the end of that first year I noticed something else. I realized that a number of the patients that I had seen, who were supposed to die within a few months, were still alive. True, they still had their disease, but they were still alive! Some of them were now up and around and participating in family activities. Some were, once more, working in their flower beds. So, again, I continued.

At this point let me interrupt the story and define the terms *"primary* cancer" and *"metastatic* cancer." *Primary* cancer is cancer in one place in the body. The usual progression of this disease is that it spreads into other areas of the body. When the disease spreads from its primary site into other areas, it is called *metastatic* cancer.

Sorry about the interruption, but it was necessary. Now, back to our story.

My biggest surprise came at the end of my third year. At that time I sat down and went through all of the records of all of the patients that I had on this nutritional program. To my amazement, I found that not one single one of the patients that I had seen with primary cancer had developed metastatic disease. With "orthodox" treatment, by this time, most of them should have. This was when I knew that I had something!

You would think that a small town doctor working with a few cancer patients and a relatively new approach to the treatment of cancer, would be ignored and left alone. Right?

W rong!

Preparing for Battle

Chapter Four

To the best of my knowledge, there was no law in the State of Ohio which would prevent me from using Laetrile. I had checked with several attorney friends. I had asked them to see what the law was. They reported that there were no laws in the State of Ohio regarding the use of Laetrile.

I called the Ohio State Medical Association. A woman answered the phone. Our conversation went something like this:

"I would like to know the present legal status of Laetrile in Ohio."

"Laetrile is illegal," I was told.

"If Laetrile is illegal, there must be some statute which says it is illegal. Would you please give me that statute number so that my attorney can look it up for me."

"Laetrile is illegal," I was told again.

"Yes, I understand that, but what is the statute number that makes it illegal?"

"Laetrile is illegal," I was told for the third time.

"You have told me that three times now, but you have not given me the precise law that makes it illegal."

"Well, it is not approved by the FDA," was the reply this time.

"Does that make it illegal?"

"No."

"Why, then, did you tell me three times that it was illegal?"

"Because that was what I was told to say if anyone inquired about Laetrile," was her reply.

You can imagine my surprise (shock would be more like it) when, in the Fall of 1976, I received a certified letter from the Medical Board of the State of Ohio requiring me to appear, two weeks hence, before that Board for a hearing because I was using Laetrile. The first thing I did was call The Committee for Freedom of Choice in California. I do not remember with whom I spoke, but it was probably Bob Bradford. The advice I was given was to contact an attorney by the name of Mr. George Kell.

Mr. Kell was the attorney who defended Dr. John Richardson in his long and difficult legal battles with the State of California over the use of nutritional therapy and Laetrile. The story of Dr. John Richardson, and his fight for the rights of his patients to choose the type of treatment they wanted, became a best-selling book entitled *Laetrile Case Histories* . In my opinion, Dr. John Richardson is one the great heroes of medicine.

Because of his work with Dr. Richardson, George Kell was probably the most knowledgeable attorney in the country at that time on the subject of nutrition and Laetrile. I called Mr. Kell and we talked at some length. He told me some things that I should do and some things not to do. He

1. See *Laetrile Case Histories; The Richardson Cancer Clinic Experience,* by John A. Richardson, M.D., and Patricia Griffin, R.N., B.S. Originally published by American Media.

told me a number of things that my attorney should and should not do. Finally he said, "The best thing to do is for me to be there."

Among other things, Mr. Kell had recommended that, in the two weeks time that we had, we contact as many of my patients as possible and ask these patients to write to the State Medical Board on my behalf. For the next five days and nights we did exactly that. I had two telephone lines coming into my office. My office girl, Ruthie Coe, (without additional pay, bless her heart) and I would return to my office every night and make telephone calls until about 10:00 P.M. Meanwhile, Betty, having a list of her own, was making calls from our home. The response was overwhelming! I do not know how many letters actually went into the State Medical Board. I do know that there were some forty or fifty patients who were kind enough to send me copies of the letters they had written. The ground work, as directed by Mr. Kell, had been laid.

The hearing was scheduled for a Thursday morning. George Kell arrived at the Columbus, Ohio airport about 10:30 P.M. the night before. Until the wee hours of the morning we stayed up and discussed strategy. Mr. Kell explained to me that he would attempt to make the Medical Board angry at him, thus taking their anger away from me.

During the hearing, Mr. Kell was extremely successful in doing just that. On at least four occasions he said to the members of the Board, "If you decide to take this matter to court, you will have me to deal with." As things turned out, it became obvious that the Medical Board of the State of Ohio did not wish to deal with Mr. George Kell. For his wonderful performance, I am eternally grateful to him.

ALIVE AND WELL

For those who are wondering how much it cost to bring in an attorney from California to defend me, let me say that Mr. Kell's charge was *extremely* reasonable. He charged me only for his air fare (coach, of course) and for his time before the Medical Board. This came to about $700. There are still some people on this earth to whom principle is more important than money. George Kell is one of those people.

Several months went by before I heard anything from the State Medical Board. Then, an Enforcement Officer of the Board, as he called himself, appeared in my office without an appointment and insisted that I see him immediately. As soon as I finished with the patient at hand, I did see him. He wanted to know if I was still using Laetrile. I assured him that I was. He told me that the Medical Board wanted to take away my medical license. I told him I knew that, but, in order for them to do so, they would have to go through the courts. I told him I would insist on a jury trial, and that I would parade before the jury all of the patients who had written letters to the Medical Board. He said, "Oh, no, no, no! We don't want to get involved in anything like that." I assured him that was exactly what the Board would become involved in, and that they would again be confronted by Mr. George Kell.

At this point he backed down. We discussed a few irrelevant things. Then he said, "I just want you to know that the State Medical Board is not happy with what you are doing." I said to the Enforcement Officer, "I was not placed on this earth to please the State Medical Board. I was placed on this earth to please God. I know that the nutritional program I am using adds far more to the quality and quantity of life of the cancer patient than anything offered by orthodox medicine. Therefore, I am obligated to God to do what I know to be right. Whether the State

Medical Board agrees or disagrees is not important. It is important *only* that I do what pleases God, because, at my death, I will be judged by God and not by the State Medical Board."

Except for a letter in 1978, that was the last that I heard from the Medical Board of the State of Ohio for fourteen years (until 1990). I'll tell you about that later.

The Battle Begins

Chapter Five

My first confrontation with the FDA came when Patrick Mahoney, a long time friend, who was then working for Birch Research Corporation, contacted me. Part of Patrick's job was to review all major newspapers and government documents and to file any information which may at sometime be of any news value. Patrick had run across a notice in the *Federal Register* which said that there were going to be Administrative Hearings on Laetrile in Kansas City, Missouri, on May 2-3, 1977. According to the notice, anyone who wished to speak for or against Laetrile was to write to the given address and ask for time to present testimony. At Patrick's urging, I wrote to that address and asked for fifteen minutes.

I really had no idea what this was all about. But, by this time, I had three years of experience using Laetrile as a part of a total nutritional program. I knew that it was part of what was necessary to improve the quality and quantity of life of many cancer patients. Again, I felt that I had a moral obligation to present my findings at that Administrative Hearing, so Betty and I went. It wasn't until after we got there that I fully understood what was going on.

In early 1977, Mr. Glen L. Rutherford from Oklahoma City developed cancer. He chose to go to Mexico for the treatment of his cancer because they were using a nutritional program that included Laetrile. A few weeks later, when Mr. Rutherford returned to the United States, his Laetrile was confiscated when he crossed the border. This was done by Government order. Mr. Rutherford then filed suit in Federal Court against Joseph A. Califano, Secretary of Health, Education and Welfare and against Donald Kennedy, Commissioner of the Food and Drug Administration *et al.* for the right to have his Laetrile. This I know to be true because I have the court record. What follows I do not know to be true because I was not there, but I will relate the story to you as it was told to me by those who were there.

The trial between Mr. Rutherford and the Government went on for several weeks. Federal Judge Luther Bohanon presided. Each day the FDA attorneys would tell the court that the FDA had hundreds and hundreds of studies that proved that Laetrile would not work. Toward the end of the trial Judge Bohanon said to the FDA attorneys, "Tomorrow, when you come into court, I want you to bring with you all of these studies that have been done by the FDA on Laetrile."

The following morning, when the trial began again, the Judge asked for the studies. The FDA attorneys said, "Your Honor, we did not bring the studies because they are so scientific that we don't think you can understand them." This, as you can well imagine, did not please the Judge. He insisted that all of the studies must be in his court room the following morning.

The next morning there were no studies. When the Judge asked why, the FDA attorneys said the studies were so voluminous they were not sure that all of the studies would fit in his court room. The Judge then stated that, if necessary, he would empty the entire court house, *but* he wanted all of those studies in his court the following morning.

The following morning there were no studies. Again, the Judge asked why. The FDA attorney said very simply, "Because, Your Honor, there are no studies." Of course, the Judge was irate. The FDA attorneys explained that each evening after the trial they would call Washington. Each evening the Washington office of the FDA would assure the attorneys that they had all of these studies. When the attorneys finally pinned down the Washington office, they said that they had done no studies at all on Laetrile. This was when Judge Bohanon called for Administrative Hearings.

In truth, as time has gone on, I have found much evidence to make me believe that the FDA had, indeed, done a great many studies on Laetrile. The problem was they apparently had found that—when properly used with other vitamins, minerals, enzymes and diet—Laetrile could be very beneficial to many cancer patients. There was no way the FDA was going to admit this! For more than fifteen years they had been saying that Laetrile was of no value. To come out now and say that they had been wrong was unthinkable. The fuss and furor that would have come from the people of this country would have been tremendous. Congress, rapidly, would have been forced to do away with the FDA. To the government, this would have been a terrible loss. After all, the "most important" function of any government bureaucracy is to perpetuate itself. It is my opinion, and only an opinion, that it was easier for the FDA to say that they had done no studies than to reveal what their studies had actually shown. It was far less dangerous to go through Administrative Hearings than to admit that they were wrong.

ALIVE AND WELL

These Administrative Hearings were something else. Of the perhaps two hundred to three hundred people who were there, almost all were pro-Laetrile. There were, of course, many doctors from the FDA who testified against Laetrile. The thing I remember most about these hearings was that, shortly before I testified, a doctor from the FDA testified that if you open a vial of Laetrile, it must be done in a large room with all of the windows open and that everyone in the room must wear a gas mask. Otherwise, he said, everyone would die from the cyanide fumes from that vial of Laetrile. Shortly thereafter I testified that I had opened some four thousand vials of Laetrile. I stated that I had opened them in a small room with all of the windows closed and that neither I, nor any of my staff, had worn a gas mask. I assured the Administrative Judge that I, and all of my staff, were alive and quite well.

The Administrative Judge was sitting to my right and behind me. I could not see him while I was testifying. According to those in the audience who could see him, he obviously became quite angry and turned very red in the face. He had allowed some of those testifying for the FDA to run overtime with their testimony. Just as soon as my time was up, he banged his gavel and said sternly, "Your time is up!" I assured him that I would be finished in less than a minute. Down came the gavel again, and again he said angrily, "Your time is up!" I had a typewritten copy of my full testimony, which I then gave to the recording secretary. All of my testimony did appear in the full record.

The full testimony of everyone who took the stand at this Administrative Hearing was sent to Judge Bohanon. He then went through all of this material. On December 5, 1977, he rendered his final decision in the case of Rutherford vs. United States of America, Joseph A.

THE BATTLE BEGINS

Califano, Secretary of Health, Education and Welfare; Donald Kennedy, Commissioner of the Food and Drug Administration *et al.* For those of you who have access to law libraries this will be found in THE UNITED STATES DISTRICT COURT FOR THE WESTERN DISTRICT OF OKLAHOMA, No. CIV-75-0218-B.

Parts of Judge Bohanon's decision are as follows:

> The action of the Commissioner of Food and Drugs dated July 29, 1977, is declared unlawful and such action, findings and conclusions are hereby vacated, set aside and held for naught.
>
> The Secretary of Health, Education and Welfare and his subordinates in the Food and Drug Administration are hereby permanently enjoined and restrained from interfering, directly or indirectly, or acting in concert with United States Customs Service or others, with the importation, introduction, or delivery for introduction into interstate commerce by any person of Laetrile (Amygdalin)....
>
> The Secretary of Health, Education and Welfare and his subordinates in the Food and Drug Administration are hereby permanently enjoined and restrained from interfering with the use of Laetrile (Amygdalin) for the care or treatment of cancer by a person who is, or believes he is, suffering from the disease;
>
> The Secretary of Health, Education and Welfare and his subordinates in the Food and Drug Administration are hereby enjoined and restrained from interfering with any licensed medical practitioner in administering Laetrile (Amygdalin) in the care or treatment of his cancer patients.

In giving the reasons for reaching his decision, Judge Bohanon cited the testimony of many of us at the Administrative Hearing. I am proud to say that he cited my testimony on several occasions.

The result of this decision is what became known as "the affidavit system." The way this system worked was-if

43

a patient wanted Laetrile, he would have to sign an affidavit, with five copies, stating that he wanted it. He would have to give his name, address and telephone number. The doctor had to sign the same affidavit (all five copies) stating that he would administer the Laetrile. Both the patient's and the doctor's portions of the affidavit had to be notarized. This was then sent to a pharmacist who kept one copy and sent the rest to the FDA. The FDA would send the purchase order to Mexico, where the Laetrile was manufactured. The order would be filled, packaged, addressed to the patient and sent from Mexico to an FDA office in California. There it would be checked with the proper affidavit and sent to the patient. It was not at all unusual for the FDA to call the patient to make sure that he had ordered that amount of Laetrile. To some patients this was merely annoying. To many others it was very upsetting because they were made to feel that they had done something illegal.

This is where we ran into an early problem. The FDA did not want to comply with Judge Bohanon's court order. When the packaged, addressed orders were sent to California, the FDA would allow the packages to sit for many days in their office before forwarding them to the patients. A pharmacist in Baltimore, Maryland found an answer to this. His customers were complaining that they were not getting their Laetrile orders. He gave them the telephone number of Judge Bohanon's office. The customers began bombarding the Judge's office with complaints. The Judge would call the FDA, and for awhile things would run smoothly. Within a few weeks, however, the problem would again occur. The result was more phone calls to the Judge's office. The pharmacist here in Ohio, who was handling my patients, was not involved in the phone call procedure to Judge Bohanon. He did, however, receive a call from the Judge's office asking him to "call off the dogs" because the Judge would take care of the matter. Exactly what the Judge told the Commissioner of the Food and Drug Administration, Donald Kennedy, I do not know. I do know that this hold-up never happened again with any of my patients.

Judge Bohanon's decision and the affidavit system went from court to court. Many courts upheld his decision. Some courts did not. His decision and his affidavit system were finally overturned in February, 1989.

I am not sure what the status of Laetrile is in most states, but I do know what it is in the state of Ohio now. No doctor in this state may write a prescription for Laetrile, but anyone in this state who wishes to have Laetrile may obtain it without prescription. If the patient buys the Laetrile and takes it to his doctor, his doctor may then give the Laetrile to the patient. This is, of course, bureaucracy at its worst. I can buy penicillin and I can give it to a patient. But, I cannot buy Laetrile and give it to a patient. The patient can buy the Laetrile and bring it to me, and then I can give it to him.

Anyway, in the state of Ohio, the patient can get Laetrile and the doctor can give it to him in the proper manner and the proper dosage. I thank God for small favors!

Laetrile and Cyanide

Chapter Six

In Chapter Five I mentioned the testimony of a doctor from the FDA who said that Laetrile contains "free" hydrogen cyanide and, thus, is toxic. Somewhere in this book I wanted to correct that misconception. Perhaps this is the best time to do so.

There is no "free" hydrogen cyanide in Laetrile. As pointed out in Chapter Two, when Laetrile comes in contact with the enzyme beta-glucosidase, the Laetrile is broken down to form two molecules of glucose, one molecule of benzaldehyde and one molecule of hydrogen cyanide (HCN). Within the body, the cancer cell—and only the cancer cell—contains that enzyme. The key word here is that the HCN must be FORMED. It is not floating around freely in the Laetrile and then released. It must be manufactured. The enzyme beta-glucosidase, and only that enzyme, is capable of manufacturing the HCN from Laetrile. If there are no cancer cells in the body, there is no beta-glucosidase. If there is no beta-glucosidase, no HCN will be formed from the Laetrile.

It is worthwhile repeating something I said in Chapter Two: In 1977 it was thought that the hydrogen cyanide formed in the above-mentioned chemical reaction exerted the toxic effect against the cancer cell. In the past several years there has been much evidence to show that this chemical reaction produces only a minute amount of hydrogen cyanide, that the hydrogen cyanide is quickly converted to thiocyanate and probably has little, if any, toxic effect on the cancer cell. It is the benzaldehyde formed in this chemical reaction that is extremely toxic to the cancer cell.[1]

Laetrile does contain the cyanide radical (CN⁻). This same cyanide radical is contained in Vitamin B 12, and in berries such as blackberries, blueberries and strawberries. You never hear of anyone getting cyanide poisoning from B 12 or any of the above-mentioned berries, because they do not. The cyanide radical (CN⁻) and hydrogen cyanide (HCN) are two completely different compounds, just as pure sodium (Na⁺) - one of the most toxic substances known to mankind - and sodium chloride (NaCI), which is table salt, are two completely different compounds.

If the above is true, how did the story ever get started that Laetrile contains "free" hydrogen cyanide? Guess! No, it was not G. Edward Griffin. It was the Food and Drug Administration.

I remember reading in some newspaper back in the late 1960's or early 1970's a news release from the FDA. This release stated that there were some proponents of a substance known as "Laetrile" (I'd never heard of it before) who were saying that this substance was capable of forming hydrogen cyanide in the presence of the cancer cell. The release continued by saying that, if this were actually true, we had, indeed, found a substance which was target-specific, and would be of great value to the cancer

---

1. For a more detailed analysis of the theoretical action of Laetrile against cancer cells, see G. Edward Griffin, *World Without Cancer* (Thousand Oaks, CA: American Media, 1974).

patient. But, the news release went on to say, the FDA had done extensive testing of this substance, "Laetrile," and found no evidence that it contained hydrogen cyanide or that any hydrogen cyanide was released in the presence of the cancer cell. Thus, they said, Laetrile was of no value.

When it was clearly established some time later that Laetrile did, indeed, release hydrogen cyanide in the presence of the cancer cell, how do you suppose the FDA reacted? Did they admit that they were wrong? Did they admit that they had done a very inadequate job in running their tests? No! They now proclaimed that Laetrile contained hydrogen cyanide and thus was *toxic!*

So, here is a bureau of the Federal Government which, a short time before, had said that the reason Laetrile did not work was because it did not release hydrogen cyanide in the presence of cancer cells. Now, when they find that it does, they say that it is toxic. When offered an opportunity to present evidence of Laetrile's toxicity in Federal Court, they admitted that they had none. (See Chapter One)

When anyone tells you that Laetrile contains "free" hydrogen cyanide, that individual is either mis-informed or wants to mis-inform you.

Debunking the Debunkers

Chapter Seven

Between the years 1975 and 1980 there were so many things happening that I am sure I do not remember all of them. Some of them were going on at the same time. These stories need to be told. While the exact chronological order of these stories may be incorrect, the stories are true.

Certainly one story that needs to be told is that of Dr. Kanematsu Sugiura. In 1975, Dr. Sugiura was, and had been for some years, one of the most respected cancer research scientists at Sloan-Kettering. In working with cancerous mice, Dr. Sugiura found that, when he used Laetrile on these mice, seventy-seven per cent of them did not develop a spread of their disease (metastatic carcinoma). He repeated this study over and over for two years. The results were always the same. Dr. Sugiura took his findings to his superiors at Sloan-Kettering, but his study was never published. Instead, Sloan-Kettering published the results of someone else who claimed that he had used Dr. Sugiura's protocol. This "someone else's" study showed that there were no beneficial effects from the use of Laetrile. Dr. Sugiura complained. He was fired. A book was written about all of this entitled *The Anatomy of A Cover-up*. This book has all the actual results of Dr. Sugiura's work. These results do, indeed, show the benefit of Laetrile. Dr. Sugiura stated in this book, "It is still my belief that Amygdalin cures metastases." Amygdalin is, of course, the scientific name for Laetrile.

A few months later, a cancer researcher at Mayo Clinic, in a private, informal conversation with a friend of mine, stated that it was very unlikely that any positive effects from the use of Laetrile would ever be published because "the powers above us want it that way."

During this period of time, the National Cancer Institute (NCI) stated that it wanted to run a study to show the difference between patients treated with orthodox therapy (surgery, radiation, chemotherapy) and those treated with nutritional therapy. I was asked to participate in this study. I went to New York to meet with one of the doctors who was conducting the study. I will call him Dr. Enseeye (not his real name, of course). There was a group of perhaps six or seven of us who had dinner that night with Dr. Enseeye. Betty and I were seated next to him.

Dr. Enseeye explained the study to me. The NCI would take a group of cancer patients and treat them in the orthodox method. Those of us who were using nutritional therapy would take a similar group of patients and treat them by our method. The NCI would then compare the results. This is the conversation that followed:

"What will the NCI use as a criteria for success or failure in these treatments?" I asked.

"Tumor size," Dr. Enseeye replied.

I said, "Let me make sure I understand what you are saying. Suppose you have a patient with a given tumor. Let's suppose that this patient is treated by one of these two methods. Let's say that the tumor is greatly reduced in size in the next three months, but the patient dies. How will the NCI classify that?

"The NCI will classify that as a success"

52

DEBUNKING THE DEBUNKERS

"Why?" I asked.

"Because the tumor got smaller," he replied.

I then asked, "Suppose you have a similar patient with a similar tumor who was treated with a different method. Suppose that after two years this patient is alive and well, but the tumor is no smaller. How will the NCI classify this?"

"They will classify that as a failure."

"Why?" I asked.

"Because the tumor did not get any smaller," he said. Dr. Enseeye went on to say, "In this study the NCI will not be interested in whether the patient lives or dies. They will be interested only in whether the tumor gets bigger or smaller."

I chose *not* to participate in this study!

During this period, the FDA was sending speakers throughout the country to talk about the "evils" of Laetrile. One such speaker was scheduled to appear on the campus of Macalester College in St. Paul, Minnesota in the spring of 1978. It just so happened that my son Rick was a sophomore at Macalester College at that time. Rick was very knowledgeable on the subject of Laetrile. When he found out when the talk was to be given, he called his older brother, Bill, who was a senior at the University of Wisconsin in LaCrosse. Bill was equally knowledgeable about Laetrile and agreed to come to Macalester for the speech. Rick had also recruited a friend who was a freshman at his school, Michelle Kleinrichard, who knew as much about the subject as the two of them.

The three of them went to the speech, but they did not sit together. Bill sat near the center just beyond half-way back in the auditorium. Rick sat toward the front on the right. Michelle sat toward the front on the left.

ALIVE AND WELL

According to all three of them, the speaker left much to be desired. It was easy to see he had been given the speech to read, and that he had only a superficial knowledge of the subject. At the end of the speech he asked for questions. The first one on his feet was Bill (in the center). What happened was as follows:

Bill: "You said that you knew of a patient who had cancer and was treated with Laetrile. You said that the patient died, and this proved that Laetrile was worthless. Hubert Humphrey had cancer and was treated with chemotherapy. He died three months ago. Doesn't that prove that chemotherapy is worthless too? But, that's not my question. You also said that a little girl in New York took five Laetrile pills and died from cyanide poisoning. The parents now state that she took only one Laetrile pill. She was fine for three days. Then the doctors started treating her for cyanide poisoning. The next day she died. How do you explain this?"

Speaker: "I have no explanation for this."

Bill: "Another question."

Speaker: "No, we'll go to someone else."

With this, the speaker turned to another nice looking young man on his left. This other nice looking young man was Rick. (I have to say they were "nice looking" because I'm their father.) Rick pointed out that the speaker had stated that work done by Dr. Harold Manner, using Laetrile alone, had shown no positive results on cancerous mice. This, the speaker had said, was considered to be of great scientific value. Subsequent work done by Dr. Manner using Laetrile in combination with pancreatic enzymes and Vitamin A had shown excellent results. Yet, the speaker had indicated that these latter results were of no scientific value. Rick's question was why were these latter results ignored. The speaker could not answer that question.

The speaker then turned to his right. There, standing and smiling at him, was a pretty young lady. The speaker must have thought, "At last, a friendly face." The young lady was Michelle. Michelle was a member of the debate team at Macalester. The speaker was badly out-classed. She hit him with both barrels. She asked for a full explanation of why, if so many people die from chemo-therapy, is chemotherapy so good? Why, if Laetrile makes people feel better, is Laetrile so bad? She asked who determined that Dr. Manner's recent results were not scientific. The poor speaker was in trouble. He hemmed and hawed, but never answered her questions. Finally, he said, "The question and answer period is over." He turned and rapidly left the stage. In five minutes Bill, Rick and Michelle had completely destroyed the credibility of the forty-five minute speech.

So, you ask, whatever became of those three free-thinking undergraduates who perpetrated this dastardly deed on this unsuspecting FDA speaker? (You probably weren't going to ask, but I'm going to tell you anyway!).

Bill got his law degree from Capital University in Columbus, Ohio. He worked for Congressman Lawrence P. McDonald as his legislative director until the KAL Flight 007 incident. Subsequently, he worked for Congressman Al McCandliss as his legislative director. Later, he became the Republican counsel for the House Banking Committee. He has since gone to work for a private business.

Rick got his Ph.D. in Astronomy from the University of Texas. He is a professor of astronomy at the Massachu-setts Institute of Technology. Rick was, incidentally, the first astronomer to view the moon around the planet Pluto.

ALIVE AND WELL

The International Astronomical Society has named an asteroid (a small planet), Asteroid 2873 Binzel, in his honor. In 1982, Rick and Michelle were married.

Michelle, in addition to being a full-time housewife and a full-time mother of two children, has also managed to complete her Ph.D. in Business Management. When those two children become teenagers, Michelle is going to need all of her debating skills. I don't know anything about business management, but as the father of six children, I sure do know about debating. I wish I had taken it in college.

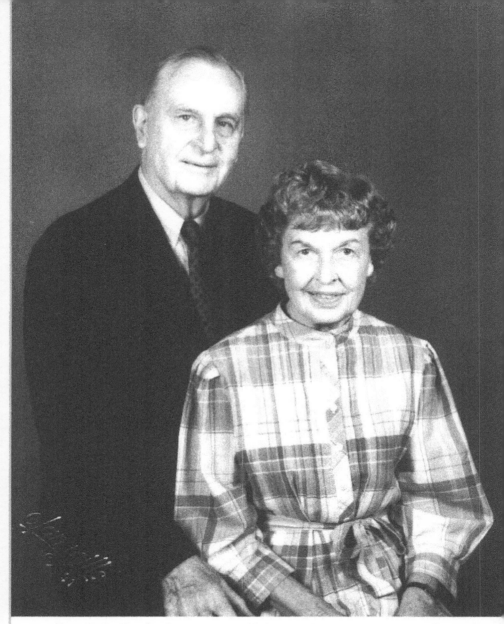

Mrs. Polly Todd, shown here with her husband, Jack, was told that her chances of surviving her breast cancer were slim. She rejected chemotherapy and radiation and began nutritional therapy instead. Twenty years later, she is still alive and well. (Case #1)

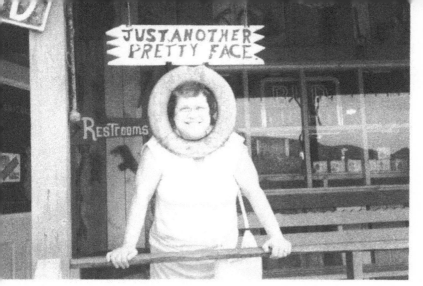

Above: Sue Tarbutton's breast cancer was discovered in 1983. She decided against surgery and choose nutritional therapy. She is shown here enjoying a full life more than ten years later. (Case #2)

Below: Elizabeth Winschel, shown here with her children and grandchildren, was diagnosed in 1976 as having colon cancer with malignant cells also in the abdomen. For over 17 years she has received nutritional therapy and has lived a normal life. (Case #3)

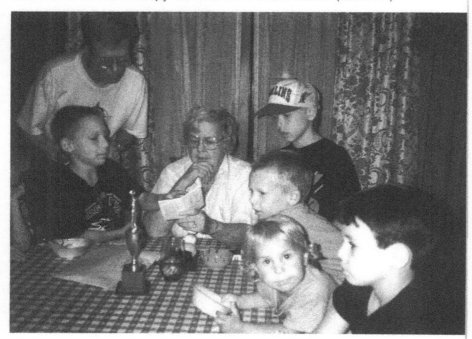

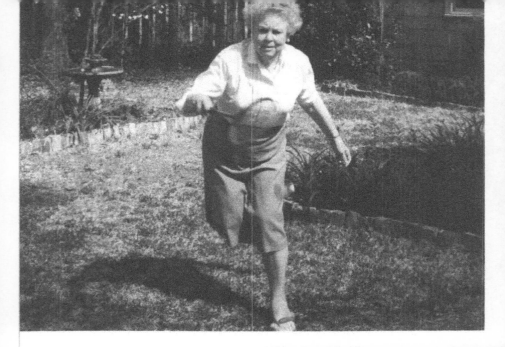

Above: Beverly Batson had half of her stomach removed in 1988 because of cancer. Then she went on nutritional therapy without radiation or chemotherapy. She is now 75 years old and has had no reoccurrence. (Case #5)

Right: Wasley Krogdahl was diagnosed in 1978 as having carcinoma of the urinary bladder. Several tumors were removed and he started nutritional therapy. Fifteen years later, at age 75, he has had no return of his cancer. (Case #4)

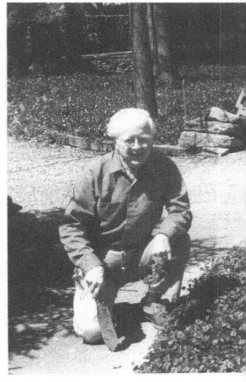

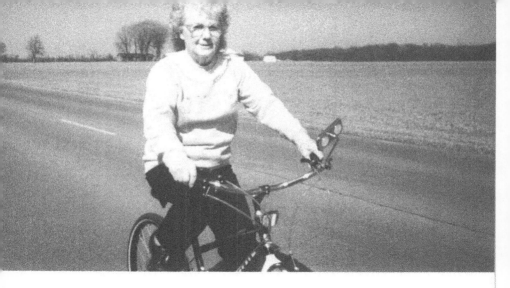

Above: Pauline Wilcox had a breast removed in 1983. When she stopped her nutritional therapy, the cancer returned in 1988. Now that she has returned to the program, she is in excellent health. (Case #10)

Below: Jean Henshall contracted myeloma (cancer of the bone) in 1986. She began nutritional therapy in 1987 and, although her response was slow at first, she is now in excellent health. (Case #6)

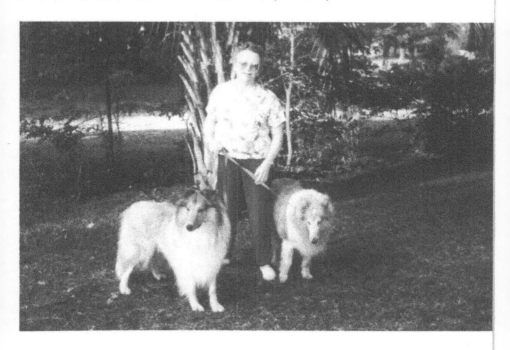

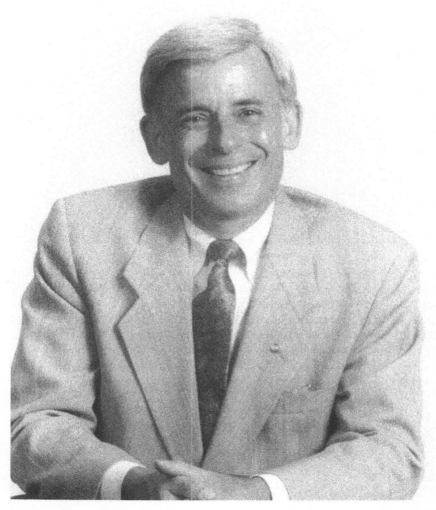

Above: Rex Perry chose not to have radiation for his malignant lymphoma. He now has been on nutritional therapy for 15 years and has has no further problems with his disease. (Case #9)

Next page, top: Irene Dirks developed cancer of the uterus in 1981. A hysterectomy was done and she started nutritional therapy. Fourteen years later, at age 73, she is healthy and active. (Case #13)

Next page, bottom: Connie Stork developed a malignant tumor of the brain in 1970, which was partially removed. After receiving radiation, another mass had to be removed, although much of the tumor remained. Her sight was damaged by the tumors and possibly the radiation. She now has been on nutritional therapy for 19 years and is blessed with a sound mind and body. (Case #11)

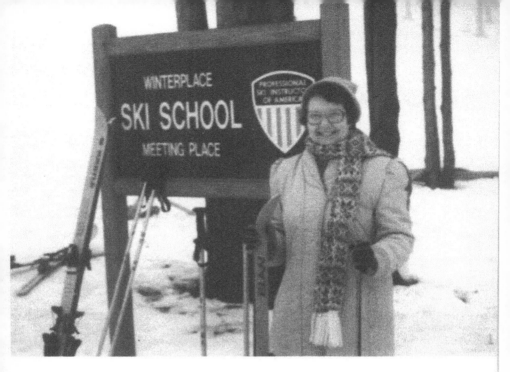

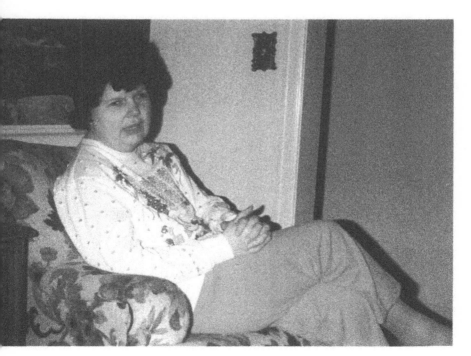

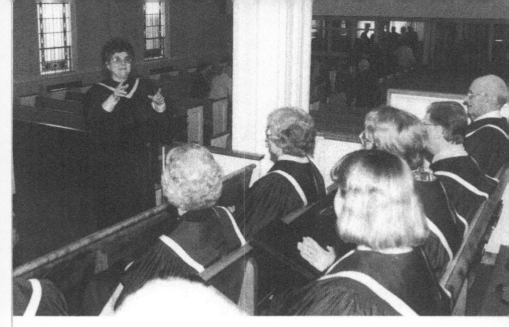

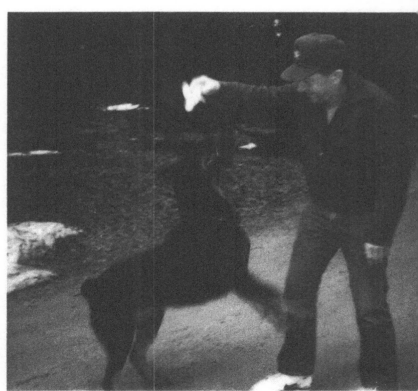

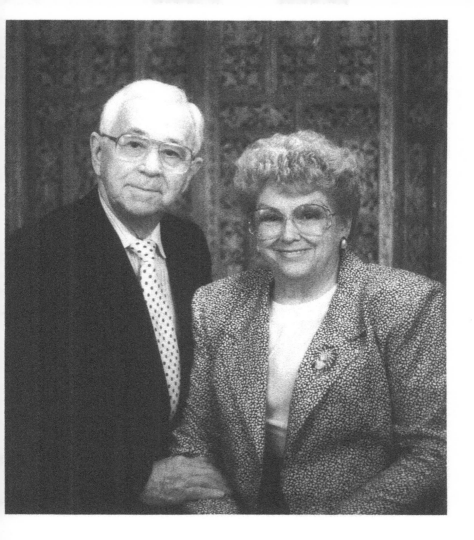

Above: Helyne Victor, shown here with her husband, Joe, began nutritional therapy after surgery for cancer of both breasts 20 years ago. She is now 74 years old and feeling great. (Case #15)

Opposite page, top: Alice Silverthorn had a breast removed in 1971 because of carcinoma. After radiation and chemotherapy the cancer spread throughout her body. She stopped chemotherapy and turned to nutritional therapy instead. Now, 18 years later, she is alive and well. (Case #19)

Opposite page, bottom: E.D. developed carcinoma of the lung in 1991. After surgery, he was put on chemotherapy which he refused to continue. X-rays showed large tumors remaining in his lung. He began nutritional therapy in 1992. By 1993, x-rays showed the tumors were gone. (Case #21)

The Joey Hofbauer Story

Chapter Eight

One Tuesday night about eight o'clock, in late November, 1978, I received a telephone call from Professor Francis Anderson, a professor at the Albany School of Law in Albany, New York. Professor Anderson told me that he was representing an eight-year-old boy, Joey Hofbauer, who had been diagnosed as having Hodgkins Disease (a form of cancer of the lymph nodes). He told me that the Saratoga County Department of Social Services was trying to force the parents to allow the use of chemotherapy in the treatment of his disease. The parents did not want the child to have chemotherapy because they had already begun to have him treated with nutritional therapy. Professor Anderson explained that there was to be a court hearing on the following Thursday. He wanted to know if I would be willing to come to Albany and testify on the boy's behalf. I told him that I would.

The Professor then stated that the family did not have much money and asked me how much I would charge. I told him that I would charge nothing for coming. Professor Anderson said, "That's wonderful, because I am not charging them anything for my services either." I told him that, if they could afford to pay my expenses, that would be fine, but if they couldn't, I'd pay my own way. He assured me that paying my expenses would be no problem for them.

I arrived in Albany about 10:30 P.M. on Wednesday. I was met at the airport by Professor Anderson, Mr. John Hofbauer (Joey's father) and by two brothers, whom I will simply call Bob and Harold, who were friends of John Hofbauer. They took me to my motel, and the whole group came up to my room. It was there that I learned what had been going on. I will tell you the story as it was told to me that night.

Joey Hofbauer had been diagnosed as having Hodgkins Disease some months earlier. His doctors said that the only treatment was chemotherapy. His father, John, knew others who had taken chemotherapy. He did not want this for his son. Instead, he took Joey to a medical clinic in Jamaica for nutritional therapy.

When Joey's doctors found out that his father had not only taken him out of the country, but was also not going to have him treated with chemotherapy, they became irate. They filed a "child abuse" claim against John.

A few weeks later, when John returned to Albany with Joey, the powers-that-be were lying in wait. Less than twenty-four hours after their return, a sheriff and several deputies literally broke down the front door of the Hofbauer home and kidnapped Joey. They took him to a hospital where, according to the Saratoga County Department of Social Services, he would receive chemotherapy whether the parents approved or not.

John Hofbauer called his family attorney and explained the situation. His attorney told him that he did not want to become involved in a case of this nature. John then took the telephone directory and called almost every attorney in Albany. The reply was always the same.

"While I sympathize with you, I do not want to become involved."

It was now about eleven o'clock at night. John had gone through all of the attorneys in Albany. Out of sheer desperation he called his friends, Bob and Harold, in Boston. Bob answered the phone. John explained what had happened and about his inability to find an attorney to represent him. Bob told him that he and Harold would meet him in Albany the next morning.

Bob and Harold drove all night and arrived at the Hofbauer home about 6:00 A.M. The battle plan was drawn. At 7:00 A.M. Bob left. He spent the entire day visiting every radio and television station in the city. He told each and every one of those stations the story of Joey Hofbauer, and that Joey's father had not been able to find an attorney who was willing to represent him. By mid-afternoon this story was on every radio station and every television station in Albany.

Watching the six o'clock news on television was Professor Francis Anderson. He immediately called John Hofbauer and told him that he would be happy to represent him, and that there would be no charge for his service. It was two hours later that Professor Anderson called me. To this day, I do not know how these people got my name. They never said, and I never thought to ask.

We were by now into the wee hours of the morning. Professor Anderson asked me if I had ever testified in a case of this nature. I told him that I had not. He took time to go over the types of questions he would be asking me on direct examination. This was not a problem at all. He then went into what I could expect on cross-examination. In the next hour, I probably learned more about court room procedure than I have ever learned since. He told me what questions I would be asked and how to handle those questions. The thing I remember most is that Professor Anderson told me that the attorneys for the other side would probably start naming a number of medical books and ask me if I had read them. He told me that if I had not read them just say, "No." He explained that the court does not expect that every doctor has read every medical book that has ever been written. If I had read the book say, "Yes." He told me that if I did say , "Yes," they would take some quote from that book and ask if I remembered that quote. If I did not remember that quote, I was to reply, "No, I do not remember that quote. My statement was that I have read the book, but I did not memorize it." This lesson, alone, has helped me through many subsequent court procedures.

When the news began to break on all of the radio and television stations, rumors began coming out of the hospital where Joey was confined. These rumors were that hospital was going to secretly transfer him to another hospital so that his chemotherapy could begin. Harold took care of that. He marched into the hospital with a cot under his arm. He went to Joey's bed and put his cot beside it. He then began to call various friends and neighbors of the Hofbauer's to set up a watch on Joey. Somebody was to be in that cot next to Joey every minute, twenty-four hours a day.

When our meeting in my motel room finally broke up, Bob and Harold told me they would pick me up at 7:00 A.M. I said that would be fine; I would be up and have had breakfast by then. They informed me I could not do that. They told me threats had been made against anyone who would testify against the medical establishment. I was told to remain in my room with the door locked until they, Bob and Harold, called for me. This seemed to be a little paranoid at the time, but I decided to just follow instructions.

At 7:00 A.M. the phone in my room rang. It was Bob calling from the lobby of the motel. He told me to look through the little peep-hole in my door. There, he said, I should see Harold. If it was not Harold, I was not to open my door but was to immediately call the motel security. I hung up the phone and looked through the peep-hole in my door. It was Harold.

The three of us had breakfast and then went to the hospital where Joey was confined. I was there to examine Joey. I was taken to the office of the hospital administrator where the necessary procedures (medical license, personal identification, etc.) were carried out. I was then turned over to another doctor who was instructed by the administrator to render me every courtesy.

When Bob, the doctor and I approached Joey's bed we were immediately challenged by a woman who occupied the cot next to Joey. Bob assured her that we were "friendly." The doctor who was assigned to me could not have been nicer. While he never let me out of his sight, he did promptly, at my request, supply me with a tongue blade and a stethoscope. I did my examination of Joey.

We went from the hospital to the court house. On the way, Bob and Harold explained to me that there would be a number of people from the newspapers and the TV stations in the lobby of the court house, and that I was not to talk to any of them. We entered the lobby of the court house. This was my first, and only, experience at seeing TV camera lights come on and having at least a dozen microphones shoved in my face at the same time. It was not a pleasant experience. Since that time I have seen this happen to others on TV at least a thousand times. I don't blame these people for getting angry at some newspaper and TV reporters. They deserve it! Somebody yelled at me, "Are you the surprise witness?" My reply was, "I don't know!"

When we got into the court room, the hearing had not begun. The Judge was there and said that any of us who were to testify could not make any statements to the media until we had completed our testimony and had been released by the Court. Bob, Harold and I spent the rest of the morning listening to the prosecution present its case. It wasn't very good. While they had a number of oncologists and pediatric specialists testify, Professor Anderson was always successful, on cross examination, in getting them to admit that they had very little success with their form of treatment. When the prosecution finished its testimony, the Judge called a lunch recess.

It was at lunch that I found out who the "surprise witness" was. It was Dr. Michael Schachter. from Nyack, New York. It is my impression that Dr. Schachter had heard about the case and had volunteered to testify on Joey's behalf. The prosecution knew I was going to testify, since they had made arrangements for me to examine Joey that morning, but apparently they did not know about Dr. Schachter. Someone must have leaked to the media that there was going to be a "surprise witness." Dr. Schachter joined us for lunch. Professor Anderson covered the same ground with him that he had covered with me the night before.

The defense began its testimony after lunch. I was the first witness. Under Professor Anderson's guidance, I gave my testimony. It was nothing extraordinary. We went through the facts that cancer was the result of a nutritional deficiency which prevented the body's immunological defense mechanisms from functioning normally. We covered the aspects of nutritional therapy and its abilities to help the body restore that normal defense mechanism. Of course, we concluded that Joey Hofbauer's chances for a better quality and quantity of life were greater with nutritional therapy than with chemotherapy.

The cross-examination was just about what Professor Anderson had said it would be. The attorneys for the County Department of Social Services used the usual attack by calling me a quack and a charlatan. This was nothing new for me. In my many debates with oncologists on TV, I had been called much worse than that. As I had learned before, and as Professor Anderson had cautioned me, "Don't let them make you angry." I just smiled. They then went into the book routine—had I read this or that book. I had read some of them. When I told them that I had read a particular book, they read some quote from the book and asked if I remembered that quote. My reply was just as Professor Anderson had coached me—"No, I don't remember that quote, but my statement was that I had read the book. I did not say that I had memorized it." This, as I best recall, concluded my testimony.

Dr. Michael Schachter followed me on the witness stand. It was the cross-examination of Dr. Schachter that I found most fascinating. Perhaps because he was a licensed physician in the state of New York, the opposing attorneys really went after him. I had never before, and have never since, seen anyone handle himself on a witness stand as well as Dr. Schachter did. I am sorry that I cannot remember the exact details of the questions asked and the answers he gave. What I do remember is that Dr. Schachter would, time after time, lead the opposing attorneys on, set a trap for them, and then at the opportune time, spring that trap. Each time he did, he would finish with a wide grin. He exhibited both his knowledge about the side effects of chemotherapy and his knowledge of nutrition. I had to leave before he was finished, but when I left, Dr. Schachter was grinning and the opposing attorneys were groaning.

I had to leave because either Bob or Harold told that it was four o'clock and that we had to catch a six o'clock flight out of here. With all the traffic, it would take at least an hour to get to the airport. Besides, we had to meet with the media outside.

I did meet with the media in the lobby of the court house. With lights glaring, I did a fifteen or twenty minute interview with the TV people. Finally, Bob and Harold said that we had to go or we'd never make it to the airport in time.

They were certainly right about the traffic. I don't remember which of the brothers was driving, but he drove like someone from Boston. I sat there most of the time with my hands over my eyes saying Hail Mary's. All I could hear was the honking of horns and the squealing of brakes from the cars beside us and behind us. Anyway, we did make it to the aiiport about a half-hour before the flight. As I walked through the terminal toward my gate, I passed one of those bars with a TV. I glanced at the TV and saw a familiar face. It was mine. I was on the five-thirty news. It was much too noisy to hear what I was saying, and I was in too much of a hurry to get to my gate to stop and listen. It's a weird feeling, though, to suddenly look up and see yourself on television.

It would be nice to say that my flight home was uneventful. This was not the case. My flight from Albany was to go to Buffalo. After a short lay-over I was to fly to Columbus. We flew into Buffalo in one of the worst snow storms I have ever seen. How that pilot was able to put that plane down on the runway, I'll never know. When I went to the desk to ask about my flight to Columbus, the clerk just laughed. He told us that was the last flight in here tonight, and there would be nothing leaving until in the morning.

The clerk made reservations for me for the 8:00 A.M. flight to Columbus and told me that the airlines would put me up in a motel for the night. When I told him my wife was waiting for me in Columbus, he assured me that we would be able to contact her. He called the airline desk in Columbus. Betty was at the desk. I explained the problem to her. She had just driven through a terrible ice storm to get to Columbus and had no desire to drive fifty miles back home again. We agreed that she should find a near-by motel, spend the night and meet my flight in the morning.

The next morning I took the motel shuttle to the airport. It was still snowing. When we got to the airport about 7:30 A.M., there was only one clerk on duty and about fifty people in line. At about 7:55 A.M. he announced that the flight to Columbus was closed and was leaving. A howl went up from the twenty-or-more of us still in line waiting to get on that flight. Bless his heart, he called back to the plane immediately and told them to hold until he could get all of the people there checked in.

It was now snowing harder than it was when I had come to the airport. The plane taxied out to the runway, gunned its engines and started its takeoff. It had trouble getting traction, sliding back and forth across the runway before finally taking off. There was a little five or six foot wooden barrier at the end of the runway. We were so low that, if I could have opened my window, I could have easily picked up that barrier. We got to Columbus without any further problems. My wife was there to meet me. Our fifty mile trip home was no joy either. We slipped and slid all of the way, but were able to stay out of most of the ditches. When I went into my office at two o'clock that afternoon, my office girl (Ruthie) asked, "How was your trip?" I thought at the time it was like someone asking Custer, when he reached the Pearly Gates, "Other than that, General, how was your day?"

At seven o'clock that night I got a phone call from Professor Anderson. The Judge had handed down his decision late that afternoon. He ruled that Joey should be returned to his parents and that he could continue to receive nutritional treatment. The Judge stated that nutritional therapy "has a place in our society" and that the parents of Joey Hofbauer were not guilty of child neglect in choosing that treatment for their son. The attorney for the State Health Department said that he was "very disappointed" with the decision.

I wish I could say that Joey Hofbauer lived happily ever after. Such is not the case. I never saw Joey again after that day, and I don't really know what happened. I do know that he was under Dr. Schachter's care for a while, and I do know that he died about two years later somewhere out of this country. Chemotherapy, I am sure, would not have prolonged his life. Hopefully, whatever was done added to the quality of his life.

The Media

Chapter Nine

At the beginning of Chapter Seven, I stated that there were many things going on in the years between 1975 and 1980. Let me, at this point, try to give you some idea of what I meant.

I was in private practice as a family physician. Although my primary obligation was to my family practice patients, I tried to take one hour in the morning and two hours in the afternoon three days a week to work with cancer patients. My waiting time for starting new cancer patients on the nutritional program was three months. This was terrible, but there were very few doctors doing nutritional therapy at that time. I was not in the office on Thursday, Saturday or Sunday. Almost all of my Thursdays were filled giving interviews, going somewhere to give a talk or to be on a television program. There were trips to Columbus, Ohio to testify before the Ohio State legislature and trips to Jackson, Michigan to testify before the Michigan State legislature. Many of my weekends were spent attending or speaking at seminars on nutrition.

Betty and our six children also needed some of my time. We had children graduating from high school, entering college and graduating from college every year during this period. The beginning and ending of the college year and college vacation time is still pretty much of a blur to Betty and me. None of our children went to the same college. Much of the time Betty would take off in one direction, and I would take off in the other to pick up, or deliver, whoever was in that direction. During this time, we also had the weddings of our oldest son and our oldest daughter.

For these reasons, I don't remember every newspaper or TV interview or even every television appearance. I would, however, like to tell you about a few which stand out in my memory.

There are some very intelligent newspaper and TV people out there. There are people like Alice Hornbaker from the *Cincinnati Enquirer.* There are people like the woman from the Akron-Canton area of Ohio, whose name I cannot remember. She had multiple sclerosis some years before and had managed, through good nutrition, to control her disease. In our interviews, both of these women understood what I meant by good nutrition and wrote excellent newspaper articles about how nutrition could help the cancer patient. There was a woman from one of the Dayton, Ohio television stations that had obviously done her homework on nutrition. My TV interview with her was delightful.

Then, there are the others. My first experience with "the other kind" was with a television station in Columbus, Ohio. This would have been in the Spring of 1977. The station had called and we had set an exact date and time for their interview. I had picked 1:00 P.M. because my office hours began at 2:00, and I figured that one hour would be sufficient time for the interview. The TV crew arrived thirty minutes late. On camera, I explained to the interviewer that Laetrile was not a miracle drug or a cancer vitamin or a cancer cure, but was just a small part of a total nutritional program. I explained that, while I could put into the body the nutritional ingredients that the body needed in order to allow its defense mechanisms to function, I had no way of knowing how efficiently that patient's body would use those nutritional ingredients. Thus, I said, I could not guarantee any patient anything. My only guarantee to the patient, I told her, was that I would do everything I could to get that patient into as good a nutritional shape as I possibly could in order to allow that patient's defense mechanisms to function as well as they possibly could.

By now, patients with 2:00 P.M. appointments were beginning to come into the office. Since we were doing the interview in my waiting room, I insisted that we move the interview to the sidewalk in front of my office. This was done. In watching the patients come into my office, the lady interviewer got the brilliant idea that the crew should film the patients in the treatment rooms while I was giving them their Laetrile injections. My reply was, "These are sick people. This is not a circus." This made her very unhappy, and she immediately concluded the interview.

Betty was there while all of this was going on. When we saw how the interview was presented on the 11:00 P.M. news that night, we were both flabbergasted. The lady interviewer did most of the talking. *Nothing* concerning the nutritional aspect of all of this, which I had so carefully gone through, was shown or even mentioned. This lady (and, perhaps, I use the term loosely) ended by saying, in a voice-over, that Dr. Binzel guaranteed that he could cure any patient with cancer.

Very early the next morning I was on the phone to the station manager. When I was finally able to get through to him, his tone was, to say the least, haughty. He just didn't have time to see me. When I suggested that it would probably take less time to see me than it would be to see my attorney, he agreed to give me an appointment. This appointment was for two o'clock that afternoon.

When Betty and I arrived for the appointment, he could not have been nicer. It seems that people from the Ohio State Medical Board had been there that morning. They watched the tape of the interview. The truth was in the tape. He was kind enough to show us the entire tape. At the end, he said that he just did not know how this woman had been able to make such a statement. He apologized for what she had done. I accepted his apology but told him that I might, because of what his station had done, be in trouble with the State Medical Board. He assured me that, if this were the case, his station would be more than happy to pay for any legal expenses that I might incur and to compensate me for any inconvenience. I never heard from the Ohio State Medical Board about this TV interview.

Perhaps the weirdest of my experiences with the media happened with a young female reporter from a Dayton, Ohio newspaper. (I'm not trying to pick on you girls. It just happened that way.) She called and made an appointment for late one Friday afternoon in the summer of 1977. I spent about two hours with her explaining nutrition and how nutrition was important in the body's defense mechanisms. I discussed Laetrile and its role in good nutrition. There was nothing unusual about the entire interview. What was unusual was the article that appeared on the front page of that Dayton newspaper on Saturday morning. There was absolutely no similarity between the article and the interview of the previous day. The article quoted me as saying that Laetrile was a miracle drug and would cure anyone's cancer. How was I so sure that there was no similarity? Because I had long been in the habit of making a tape recording of all interviews.

THE MEDIA

Early Monday morning I called my long-time friend and family attorney, John Bath, and explained the situation to him. John recommended that I first call the editor of the paper and demand a retraction. He said, "If that doesn't work, and if your tape is what you say it is, you and I may end up owning that newspaper."

I called the editor and stated my objections. He assured me that the article was probably quite correct. I then informed him about the tape recording and my conversation with my attorney. The editor promised to call me back. He did so within an hour. He told me what had happened.

The young lady who had done the interview had a date for a beach party that night. She wrote and submitted her article before she came to see me. She went from my office to her party without changing anything in her original article. The editor told me that there would be a retraction on the front page of Tuesday's paper. He was true to his word. Not only was there a full retraction, but the whole story was told. The article ended by saying that the young lady was no longer employed by the paper. John and I never got our opportunity to own a newspaper.

In 1991, a friend of mine was able to get in touch with the editor of a Columbus, Ohio newspaper. He told the editor that there was a story about the treatment of cancer that, perhaps, the paper should look into. The editor did send a young female reporter to my office. I spent several hours with her explaining why I was using nutritional therapy and telling her about the results that I had obtained. I told her that I would make all of the necessary legal arrangements which would permit someone from the paper to go through all of my patient files and verify the statistics. What I wanted was a series of articles explaining nutritional therapy and showing the results that could be obtained by its use. I told her it was not necessary that my name ever appear in the articles. What I wanted was to get this information to the public.

The young lady understood exactly what I wanted to do. However, she said her paper was an "establishment" newspaper, and it would rarely print anything with an opposing view. What I wanted to do, she explained, would be an attack on the medical establishment. She didn't think her editor would allow that. She promised she would talk with her editor about it and would contact me again only if he said, "Yes." (Don't call me. I'll call you.) She never called.

My last contact with the TV media was in July, 1993. A TV station from Columbus called and wanted to set up an interview. We set up a date and time. The interview was to be done in my home. When the crew arrived, the interviewer wanted to start filming immediately. I refused. I told her that we would not start filming until I said so. I spent the next forty-five minutes explaining what nutritional therapy was and why I was using it. I went through the whole routine of Laetrile, pointing out that, while it was an important part of nutritional therapy, it was only a small part of the total program.

She said, "Now can we film?" I told her that we would not film until we had gone through the questions that she was going to ask. She told me that she did not have any prepared questions and would just ask questions off the top of her head. She lied.

As soon as the camera began to roll, she turned to a page in her note book which was filled with prepared questions. Her first question was, "I assume from what you have said that you are the conduit for the transportation of Laetrile through the state of Ohio?" In my previous forty-five minute discussion with this woman, I had already told her that I had nothing to do with the buying, selling or distribution of Laetrile.

Her next question was, "How much do you charge for your services?" I told her that, in all of the years that I had seen cancer surgeons, oncologists and radiologists on TV, I had never heard anyone ask them what they charged for their services. I went on to explain that I discuss my charges only with the patient, not with TV people.

There were several more questions about Laetrile, and then she said, "We want to take pictures of your patient files." I told her that this would be illegal, and that I would not even consider it. She said that unless she could see those files, she would not be convinced that any such files existed. I replied, "I couldn't care less whether you're convinced. You are not going to see my files." After she had left, I thought my reply should have been, "Well, I don't think you're wearing any underwear, and I won't be convinced unless you show me." I'm so glad I didn't think of that until after she was gone!

That night on the TV news, less than a minute or a minute and a half was given to this interview. She did most of the talking. Nothing was said about nutrition. Her final comment was, "Dr. Binzel says that he has had good results with his treatment, but he has no proof." I understand why so many people distrust the media.

Re-Enter the
State Medical Board

Chapter Ten

After my 1976 confrontation with the Ohio State Medical Board, I heard nothing from them until September, 1978. I then received the following letter:

Dear Dr. Binzel:
We understand that you may be treating a patient with Laetrile who has Hodgkins Disease. Further, we understand that the patient has been diagnosed as being at least 50 to 60 per cent curable with current accepted treatment.
As you know, the use of Laetrile has been extremely controversial and has been under review by the Courts. We would appreciate your comments with respect to this matter.

Very truly yours,
William J. Lee
Administrator

My reply to this was as follows:
Dear Mr. Lee:
In response to your letter of September 27th, it would be necessary to know the name of the patient to whom you refer before I can comment on the treatment that is being used.

ALIVE AND WELL

I am quite aware that Laetrile has been reviewed by the courts. I am also aware that the legal status of Laetrile is covered by Federal Court Order # CIV -75 -0218-B, April 8, 1977, of Federal Judge Bohanon of Oklahoma City.

Sincerely,
Philip E. Binzel, M.D.

Federal Court Order #CIV-75-0218-B was the legal name of the Federal Court Order by Judge Bohanon which set up the affidavit system described in Chapter Five. Again, what this said was that any patient who wanted Laetrile could have it, and any doctor who chose to give it could do so, *if* the patient would sign an affidavit stating that he wanted it and the doctor would sign the same affidavit stating that he would give it. This Federal Court Order went on to say that any attempt by the FDA to prevent any patient from obtaining Laetrile, or any attempt by any State Medical Board to prevent any doctor from using Laetrile, would be considered contempt of court.

As seen in my letter, I did not outline these facts to the Medical Board. My thought was, "I'll give them the legal number and let them look it up for themselves."

Would you believe that I never received a reply to my letter?

It wasn't until January 30, 1990, that my next conflict with the Ohio State Medical Board began. On that date, in the middle of my office hours, a man walked into my office, handed Ruthie his card and demanded she let him see me *now*. On his card it stated that this man was an Enforcement Officer of the Ohio State Medical Board. From my previous experience with these people, I had him cool his heels until I got a break in my schedule. The "Enforcer," as he shall henceforth be referred to, told me that he had been sent to my office by the State Medical Board to immediately pick up a list of all of the patients that I had treated with Laetrile in the past five years. I told him that it was illegal for me to give anyone the name, address, telephone number or any information whatsoever about any patient without that patient's written consent. I explained that I would have to go through my records and contact each patient individually. This, I said, would take a considerable period of time. He left saying that he would be back in a few weeks.

During my conversation with the Enforcer, he volunteered the information that this investigation was probably started by a complaint from the Food and Drug Administration. He then added, "The Medical Board certainly wants to stay out of any trouble with the FDA." After thinking about this statement for a while, I began to realize how strange this whole thing was. After all, since 1977 all of the patients for whom I had prescribed Laetrile had gotten their Laetrile through the affidavit system. This meant that the FDA already had the names, addresses and telephone numbers of all such patients for the past five years. If it was the State Medical Board that wanted this information, it could easily be obtained from the FDA. The thought then dawned on me that it was possible that this investigation had nothing to do with names and addresses, but was merely for the purpose of harassment. Nothing that transpired afterwards caused me to change my mind.

That night I called my son Bill, the attorney. I told him what had happened. He said that, while he had worked only in Washington D.C. since passing the Ohio Bar exam, he still had all of his Ohio law books and would research this for me.

Within a few days I received a letter from Bill. In this letter, he quoted the exact sections of Ohio law dealing with this subject. The law said that any doctor who gave any information about any patient to anyone without that patient's written consent would have his license revoked. It went on to say that any third party who attempted to obtain such information was also in violation of the law.

Bill advised me that, since this was a verbal request and not a written request, I would be in violation of the law if I complied. Furthermore, he said, the law requires that the patient make an "informed consent." In order for the patient to do this, there were certain things the patient had to know, such as:

1. The specific nature and purpose of the inquiry.
2. Who originated the inquiry?
3. What will be done with the information provided?
4. Will I be contacted? If so, in what manner?
5. What specific information do you want from me?
6. Am I under any obligation to respond to the request?
7. Will this information be made public or used in such a way that it may be subject to becoming public?

Bill put all of this and a lot of other legal language in a letter he composed for me to send to the Medical Board. All I had to do was copy that letter, fill in the proper names and dates and send it to the President of the Medical Board. This I did. No reply to that letter was ever received.

About one month later the "Enforcer" was back. He used the usual routine— no appointment, came in the middle of my office hours, stated that he was from the State Medical Board and wanted to be seen *now*! Again, I had him wait awhile. He told me he was here to pick up the list of the patient's names and addresses that he had requested the time before. The dialogue that ensued was something like this:

Me: I don't have a list. I never got a reply to my letter.
Enforcer: What letter?
Me: The letter I sent to the President of the Medical Board.

RE-ENTER THE STATE MEDICAL BOARD

Enforcer: I don't know anything about any letter, but they never tell me anything anyway.

I showed him a copy of my letter and then asked him if he realized that, because there was nothing in writing, what he was doing was illegal. This puzzled him, so I read him the section of Ohio law which said that a third party requesting such information was in violation of the law. He said, "Gosh, I didn't know that! What are they trying to do to me up there?" He left with a very concerned look on his face.

On March 29, 1990, I received a subpoena from the Ohio State Medical Board requiring that by April 19, 1990, I provide for them the names, addresses and telephone numbers of all the patients that I had treated with Laetrile in the past five years. It was obvious that I needed a local attorney. My family attorney, John Bath, had retired, so I called Judge Evelyn Coffman. Evelyn and I had been friends for many years. She had served on the bench as Judge of the Court of Common Pleas for twenty-four years. When she left the bench, she went into the private practice of law. Bill knew her quite well and said that he would be happy to work with her in any way she wanted. I could not have made a better choice.

When Evelyn read the subpoena, she recognized immediately that it was deficient. The subpoena stated that it was issued "because of the following charges." But, there were no charges listed. Evelyn called the State Medical Board, which said it did not know what the charges were because they had been issued by the Attorney General's office. She called the Attorney General's office, and what she got mostly was the run-around—"So-and-so is handling that, and he's not here. He'll call you back." Of course, he never did. Evelyn, because of her years on the bench, had some good connections in the Attorney General's office. It didn't take her long to cut through all of this red tape. She soon got to the individual who was handling this case. She told him that the charges against her client were not listed on the subpoena and that she wanted to know what they were. He said, "They are secret." She explained that as my attorney, she had the right to know what I had been charged with. His reply was that he had orders not to tell anyone.

A few days later Evelyn was able to get in touch with someone else in the Attorney General's office. She explained to this individual that it would be impossible for me to go through all of my records and get the information they wanted by April 19. She also stated that she had serious doubts about the legality of what the Medical Board was doing and needed time to research the law. She then informed him that, if the Attorney General's office insisted on the April 19th date, her client was quite willing to take the matter to court. Judge Coffman had spoken the magic word.

I had told Evelyn during our very first conference that I was not going to give in on this unless we took it to court and lost. I really wanted to take it to court immediately, but her cooler head prevailed. As soon as she said "court" to this individual, he backed off. He agreed to give us as much time as we needed and sent her a letter to that effect.
We had won Round One!

When I first consulted Evelyn, she told me that from here on I was not to see, talk with or have any contact with any Enforcer from the State Medical Board. Should one appear at my office for any reason, he was to be sent to her office. As expected, one such Enforcer did appear in my office on April 19th, the date stated on the subpoena. He used the same unannounced, belligerent, approach as those who preceded him. I went out to the waiting room to see him. Our conversation went like this:

Enforcer: I'm here to get the list of patients.

Me: I have been advised by my attorney that, whatever you want, you are to see her.

Enforcer: I want the list. Does she have it?

Me: I have been advised by my attorney that, whatever you want, you are to see her. Her name is Judge Evelyn Coffman and this is her address. Now, let me give you some friendly advice. Don't go busting into her office like you have done here. She was a Common Pleas judge for more than twenty years, and she's *mean*. If you go busting into her office, she'll probably have you thrown in jail.

An hour later I got a call from Evelyn. She said, "What did you say to that fellow who was in your office?" I told her. She said, "Well, I wondered. He didn't come to my office, but he called me. I could tell by his voice that he was scared to death." He had not been informed about the time extension.

We had won Round Two!

The battle then shifted. The next thing I heard was that, because I had not complied with the April 19th deadline, I must now bring the entire medical records (not just the names and addresses) of all of these patients to the Ohio State Medical Board offices in Columbus. They said that they would, as time allowed, make copies of these records and send the copies to me. You can imagine my response to this! Evelyn called them and explained that:

> **1. Because of the sheer weight of these records, it would be physically impossible for me to bring them to Columbus.**

2. Because I was either actively seeing most of these patients, or advising them by phone or letter, not to have the patient's medical record available could endanger the health or the life of that patient.

3. If the State Medical Board insisted on this, we would take it to court.

Evelyn had, again, hit upon the magic word. They immediately backed down. After numerous conversations back and forth, it was agreed that the State Medical Board would send an investigator to my office and make copies of all of my Laetrile files. There were, however, some strings attached to this. Since I did not have a copying machine in my office, the Medical Board would have to bring its own. The Medical Board would have to pay for the space they were using in my office. The Medical Board would have to pay the expense of the office girl who was bringing them the files. The Medical Board would have to pay for the utilities used in this process. These payments were to be made *in advance* on each day that their investigator was here. If not, we would take the matter to court. Again, the magic word; and again, they backed down.

By October, 1990, the battle had shifted again. Having dropped the idea of copying my records, the Medical Board went back to trying to getting a list of the names and addresses. Because of a recent Ohio Supreme Court decision, it was Evelyn's legal opinion, with which Bill concurred, that I would probably have to supply them with the information they wanted. On October 15, Evelyn received a letter from the State Medical Board stating that an investigator from the Board would be in her office "at 10:00 A.M., on Friday, October 26, 1990, to review the list of names in compliance with the subpoena of March 29,

1990." Evelyn's reply, dated October 18, 1990, was as follows:

Dear Mr. Boatright,

In reflecting upon his responsibilities to his patients, Dr. Binzel recognizes also his responsibility to the Medical Board under the Ohio Revised Code and determines that he will compile a list of names, addresses and phone numbers as per the subpoena if the Board would be so kind as to do the following (and this would save the Board and the investigators's time going through the files):

1. Before the Board makes a contact with each patient the Board will give Dr. Binzel a ten day notice so that he might put the patient at ease as to the possibility of an investigation. This assurance Dr. Binzel would appreciate having in writing. I'm sure the Board can understand the trauma cancer patients are going through at best and that they need no further reasons of insecurity.

2. As soon as Dr. Binzel receives the foregoing documents he will have all names, addresses and phone numbers in the Board's hands within three weeks.

Sincerely,

Evelyn Coffman

This letter was written at my insistence. Why? Because, for most cancer patients, their disease is very psychologically traumatic and very personal. They don't want to discuss it with anyone. The last thing they need is to be harassed about the treatment that they decided was best for them. One elderly woman, who would have been on my list, was very timid. I knew that if some Enforcer from the Medical Board confronted her, she would have been scared to death. She would have been sure that she had committed some horrible crime. She didn't need that.

Also, I had some patients who had stressed to me that they did not want anyone else to know that they had cancer. One was a woman with three small children, whose husband had left her a few months before. This had been very traumatic for the children. She went on to say that, if the children now found out that she had cancer, it would be more than they could handle. I could visualize some blundering Enforcer from the State Medical Board knocking on her door. Assuming that one of the children answered the door, he would probably say, in a voice that could be heard for ten miles, "I want to talk to your mother about her cancer!" This would have been devastating to the patient and to her children.

I had another woman who worked in a large office. Her immediate superior knew that she had cancer, but she did not want anyone else in that office to know. Again, I could visualize some Enforcer from the State Medical Board coming into that office and saying, in front of a large office staff, "I want to talk to Mrs. So-and-so about her cancer!"

In good conscience, I simply could not allow this sort of thing to happen to any of my patients. I felt that I was morally obligated to protect those patients to the extent that the law would allow. By setting up the ten-day period, as described in the letter, I could contact the patient first. I could then explain to my patients that they were free to give any information to the Medical Board that they wanted, but that they were not obligated to give any information at all, if they so wished. This would give patients, such as those described above, an opportunity to write or call the Board and refuse permission to be contacted in any manner.

I told Judge Coffman that this was as far as I would go. I had been pushed to my absolute limits. If, for whatever reason, the State Medical Board did not agree to her letter, *in writing,* that was it! There were to be no more letters and no more phone calls. We would go to court! Evelyn concurred whole heartily.

While Judge Coffman was in the process of putting this letter together, I called my State Representative, Mr. Joe Haines, in Columbus and asked for an appointment to see him. He told me that he would be in Washington Court House on the next day on other business and would be happy to come to my house. We set a time. I called Evelyn. She said that she would be available to come and that she and Joe Haines were long-time friends.

The next day Betty and I met with Joe Haines, his wife and Judge Coffman. I briefly went through my program of nutritional therapy and why I was using it. I then went into my conflict with the Ohio State Medical Board and why I did not want to give the names, addresses and phone numbers as demanded by their subpoena. Evelyn filled Joe Haines in on the legal procedures that had transpired. Joe listened intently but said very little. He did ask Evelyn some questions about the legal aspects of this. However, he did not say, one way or the other, whether he would even look into the matter. The only statement he made was that, in his opinion, the Medical Board would be making a big mistake by taking this case to court.

At 10:00 A.M. on the morning of October 26, 1990, an Enforcer from the Medical Board showed up in Judge Coffman's office and told her secretary that he was there to pick up the list of names, addresses, and telephone numbers that had been promised. Evelyn was out of town. The secretary didn't know what he was talking about. She called my home and talked with Betty. Betty told her to look in my file and she would find a letter dated October 18th to the Board. Betty told her that no reply to that letter had been received. The secretary remembered the letter.

ALIVE AND WELL

Not having been there at the time, I can only relate to you the story as told by Judge Coffman's secretary. She said that she gave the letter to the Enforcer. He read it and asked if he could use the phone. She said that it was obvious from his conversation that the party on the other end of the line knew about the letter. The Enforcer's final comment was, "Why in the hell don't you tell *me* about these things before I come all the way down here!" With this, he slammed down the phone and left.

I have not heard from the Ohio State Medical Board since that day. I still do not know whether Joe Haines intervened on my behalf. I did see Joe at a meeting three or four months later. It was neither the time nor place to discuss this in detail. I did say to him, "Joe, I have not heard from the Medical Board since I last saw you." His only reply was, "No, and you're not going to!"

The Total
Nutritional Program

Chapter Eleven

In Chapter Two, I discussed the work done by Drs. Krebs, Burk, Nieper, Contreras, Navarro and Sakai. Their work showed that there are numerous nutritional deficiencies which may exist within the cancer patient. The most important thing they stressed was that, unless you correct *all* of these deficiencies, you are not going to help that patient. Thus, they were talking about a *total nutritional program*. It is that *total nutritional program* which I want to discuss in this chapter.

There is an old saying in the medical profession which goes something like this: "The doctor who treats himself has a fool for a doctor and an idiot for a patient." Or, as we would say in medical school of anyone who did something dumb, "He has bilateral stupidity with metastases."

I am going to outline, *in generalities,* the treatment that I use. For any individual reading this book who decides to treat *himself* with what follows, I say, "Please read the paragraph above again, and again and again!" If you think it is bad for a doctor to treat himself, how much worse is it for someone who knows little or nothing about medicine to try to treat himself? God did not make any two of us exactly alike, thus the exact treatment must be fitted to the needs of each patient.

The whole objective of this nutritional program is to do two things:

1. To put into the body the nutritional ingredients that the body needs in order to allow its immunological defense mechanisms to function normally, and

2. To take away from the body those thing that are detrimental to the normal function of its immunological defense mechanisms.

There are three parts to this program:

1. Vitamins and enzymes
2. Nitrilosides
3. Diet

VITAMINS AND ENZYMES

1. Multiple vitamin - 1 twice daily
2. Vitamin C 1 gram - 1 twice daily
3. Vitamin E 400 units - 1 twice daily
4. Megazyme Forte (a combination of trypsin, chymotrypsin, bromalin and zinc) - 2 three times daily
5. Pangamic acid (B15) 100 mg. - 1 three times daily
6. Pro-A-Mulsion (25,000 I.U. Vitamin A per drop) - 5 drops daily.

Since vitamins are food, they should be taken with meals or immediately thereafter. It is never a good idea to take any vitamin on an empty stomach.

NITRILOSIDES

In order to supply the necessary nitrilosides I use Amygdalin (Laetrile). Laetrile is available in 500 mg. tablets and in vials (10cc-3 gms.) for intravenous use. I use both forms. The dosage that I use is as follows:

The intravenous Laetrile is given three times weekly for three weeks with at least one day between injections

THE TOTAL NUTRITIONAL PROGRAM

(Mon., Wed., Fri.). The Laetrile is not diluted and is given by straight I.V. push over a period of one to two minutes depending on the amount given.

The dosage for the intravenous Laetrile is:

1st dose 1 vial (10cc-3 gms.)
2nd dose 2 vials (20cc-6 gms.)
3rd dose 2 vials (20cc-6 gms.)
4th through the 9th doses 3 vials (30cc-9 gms.)

Following this first three weeks of I.V. injections, the patient then has one injection of 1 vial (10cc-3 gms.) once weekly for three months. If the patient notices a considerable difference in the way he feels when the injections are reduced to once weekly, the injections are increased to two or three times a week for three weeks. The dose is then reduced again to once weekly. This is repeated as often as necessary until the patient notices no difference with the reduced dosage.

The oral Laetrile is given in a dosage of 1 gram (two 500 mg. tablets) daily on the days on which the patients do not receive the intravenous Laetrile. I have them take both tablets at the same time at bedtime on an empty stomach with water. The water is important because there are some enzymes in the fruits and vegetables and in their juices which will destroy part of the potency of the Laetrile tablets while they are in the stomach. Once the stomach has emptied, this is no problem.

It should be noted that I do not start my patients on their Laetrile, either I.V. or orally, until the patients have been on their vitamins, enzymes and diet for a period of ten days to two weeks. I find that the Laetrile seems to have little or no effect until a sufficient quantity of other vitamins and minerals are in the body. Zinc, for example, is the transportation mechanism for the Laetrile. In the absence of sufficient quantities of zinc, the Laetrile does not get into the tissues. The body will not rebuild any tissue without sufficient quantities of Vitamin C, etc.

When I start the intravenous and oral dosages of Laetrile, I also begin to increase the amount of Vitamin C. I have my patients increase their Vitamin C by one gram every third day until they reach a level of at least six grams. In some patients I use more. I find that there are some patients who develop irritation of the stomach or diarrhea with the larger doses of Vitamin C. I find by increasing this by one gram every third day that, if these symptoms develop, I can reduce the Vitamin C to a level that causes no problem. I find that most of my patients tolerate the higher doses of Vitamin C very well.

On the days that my patients receive intravenous Laetrile I ask them not to take their Vitamin A. There have been some studies indicating that Vitamin A may interfere with the body's ability to metabolize intravenous Laetrile. This has not been fully proved, but I choose to have my patients not take their Vitamin A drops on the days on which they receive their intravenous Laetrile. Also, I tell my patients not to take the Laetrile tablets on the days that they receive their intravenous Laetrile. They have received intravenously as much Laetrile as the body can handle for that period of time. There are no ill effects from taking the tablets on those days, but the effect of the tablets is wasted.

The level of nitrilosides in the body can be monitored. When the body metabolizes nitrilosides, the by-product is thiocyanate. Thiocyanate levels in the blood can be measured. I find, in general, that the patients who do best are those in whom the thiocyanate level is between 1.2 and 2.5 Mg/DL. This level can be raised or lowered by increasing or decreasing the dosage of the Laetrile tablets.

THE TOTAL NUTRITIONAL PROGRAM

I do not want to leave the impression that Laetrile is the only source of nitrilosides. As stated in Chapter Two, there are some 1500 foods that contain nitrilosides. These include apricot kernels, peach kernels, grape seeds, blackberries, blueberries, strawberries, bean sprouts, lima beans, and macadamia nuts. The advantage of using Laetrile in the cancer patient is that Laetrile is a concentrated form of nitrilosides. It can raise the nitriloside level in the body (and, thus, re-establish the body's second line of defense against cancer) much more rapidly than can be done by diet alone.

DIET

The diet that I use on my patients can be summarized as follows: "If it is animal or if it comes from animal, you can not have it. (As one patient said, "If it moves, I can't eat it.") If it is not animal or does not come from animal, you can have it, but you can not cook it." I take away from my patients all meat, all poultry, all fish, all eggs, cheese, cottage cheese and milk.

The reason for such a diet goes back to Chapter Two. Remember, I said that Dr. Krebs *et al.* had found that the cancer cell had a protein lining (or covering), and that if the body dissolves that protein lining, it would kill the cancer cell. The dissolving of that protein lining, they said, is done by the enzymes trypsin and chymotrypsin, which are secreted by the pancreas. It is important to understand that it takes large quantities of trypsin and chymotrypsin to digest animal protein. Thus, the cancer patient who is eating animal protein may be using up all, or almost all, of his trypsin and chymotrypsin for digestive purposes. This leaves none of these enzymes available to the rest of the body.

The patient would be on this diet for a minimum of four months. In that period of time, I was attempting to free the trypsin and the chymotrypsin from being used up for digestive purposes and to put these enzymes back into the body in order to restore the body's first line of defense against cancer.

The reason for the fresh fruits and fresh vegetables is, again, because of enzymes. There are some enzymes in fresh fruits and vegetables which are tremendously important in good nutrition. Any temperature over 130 degrees will destroy the enzymes in the fruits and vegetables. For this reason, the fruits and vegetables may not be cooked, canned or bottled. Frozen foods from the grocery store are also prohibited because most of these frozen foods have been processed in some manner. They have either been blanched, pasteurized or sterilized so that the enzymes have been destroyed. Those who do their own home freezing are permitted to do so as long as they do not blanch the foods before they are frozen.

This means a diet that is high in salads. Salad dressings are permitted as long as the salad dressings do not contain anything which the patient may not have. Salad dressings which contain egg or sugar are not permitted. I find that many of my patients soon begin to make their own salad dressings. This is fine as long as they start with a pure vegetable oil and use no refined sugar. I do not attempt to severely limit the salt intake of my patients unless they have a medical problem which requires it. I tell them that salt may be used in moderation, but any salt that is used should be sea salt. The mineral content of sea salt is far superior to mineral content of the salt we normally use. Iodized sea salt is fine, if they need it. I encourage them to use a variety of other herbs and spices in order to vary the salad dressings so they are not eating the same thing over and over again.

The patients are not permitted anything which contains white flour or white sugar. Whole wheat flour can be used instead of white flour. In the place of sugar they can use either honey or molasses. Foods containing preservatives are kept to an absolute minimum.

The patients are encouraged to have as wide a variety of vegetables as possible. I realize that all vegetables are somewhat similar, but each vegetable, in its own way, supplies something nutrition-wise that no other vegetable has. My patients are encouraged to have, within any two-week period of time, at least some of every vegetable available at that season.

My patients are encouraged to have as wide a variety of fruits as possible, except for the citrus fruits. Oranges, lemons, grapefruit and tomatoes (Yes, tomatoes are a citrus fruit.) are not to be more than ten percent of their fruit intake. Other fruits such as apples, peaches, and pears contain far more nutrition than do the citrus fruits. My patients are also told that, except for the citrus fruits, they should eat the seeds of their fruits. Apple seeds, grape seeds, apricot kernels, peach kernels, etc. have a high nitriloside content.

With the combined fruits and vegetables, I like for my patients to have about sixty percent vegetables and about forty percent fruits. I do not require that they weigh and measure their fruits and vegetables, but ask only that they keep the vegetable intake a little higher than the fruit intake.

Protein in the diet is, of course, very necessary. However, rather than using animal protein, I use vegetable protein. Vegetable protein requires nothing in the way of the enzymes trypsin and chymotrypsin for digestion. The things that they use for their protein content can be cooked. You do not alter or harm a vegetable protein by cooking it. The things I recommended for protein are as follows:

Whole Grains

It is important that the patients read the ingredients on the labels of everything they buy. Everything labeled "Whole Wheat Bread" is not necessarily whole grain. Many of these breads contain only a small amount of whole grain and contain a large amount of white flour, white sugar and preservatives.

Whole grain cereals are permissible as long as they do not contain sugar. Most of these do contain some preservatives, but the amount is usually quite small. I do allow my patients to use some low fat milk or skim milk on their cereal. Whole wheat macaroni, noodles, spaghetti, etc. are also readily available and are good sources of protein.

Corn

This is an excellent source of protein. My patients are permitted to have corn-on-the-cob (which may be cooked), pop corn and corn meal in any form. Corn meal mush, grits and cornbread are permitted. It is necessary, in order to make cornbread, to use some egg and some milk. This is not a problem because the amounts of the egg and milk are quite small.

Buckwheat

This is high in protein. Buckwheat pancakes and pure maple syrup are excellent. Again, in order to make the buckwheat pancakes, you must use a little egg and milk. This is not a sufficient amount to cause a problem.

Butter

Butter in small amounts is permitted. Any butter that is used should be real butter rather than any margarine.

Vegetable oil hardened into a solid is detrimental to good nutrition.

Nuts

These are an excellent source of protein. This includes all nuts except the peanut. Roasted peanuts are not permitted because of an acid that is formed in the roasting. This is not true of any other nuts. Raw peanuts are permitted, but not roasted peanuts.

Dried Fruits

Dried fruits, such as dates, raisins, and figs, are excellent nutrition and provide protein.

Beans

Some vegetables, such as those in the bean family and in the *brown* rice family, cannot be eaten raw. Soup beans, lentils, split-pea, navy beans and kidney beans, are an excellent source of protein and should be an important part of this diet. Of course, they have to be cooked. Again, I repeat that anything used for its protein content may be cooked. Meals like bean soup and cornbread provide a complete protein, as would a meal of beans and brown rice.

Let me emphasize, again, the necessity of eating raw fruits and raw vegetables. Everything that can be eaten raw should be eaten raw. So many of the things we cook can be eaten raw. For example, broccoli, spinach, turnips, potatoes, and green beans can all be eaten raw.

Beverages

No milk, other than that used on cereal and in cooking, is permitted. No caffeine is permitted. This means no coffee, no Sanka, no Decaf, etc. Natural coffee substitutes are permitted along with any of the herb teas.

I keep my patients on this type of program for at least four months. It is my opinion, in twenty years of work in this field, that it takes that long to get this defense mechanism to function normally. If, at the end of the first four months, the patient is not doing as well as I would like, I continue the strict diet for as long as necessary. At the end of four months, if the patient is doing well, I then liberalize the diet. I will then allow the patient to add chicken, turkey and fish to his diet. Ninety percent of the diet at that time consists of the original strict diet plus the chicken, turkey and fish. The other ten percent of the diet may include red meats, cooked vegetables and dairy products. I caution my patients that, within any two-weeks period of time, the red meats, cooked vegetables and dairy products should never exceed more than ten percent of their total diet.

The patients are told that they also *must* stay on their vitamins, enzymes and Laetrile until the age of 130. They are instructed to call me on their 130th birthday (although I am not sure what my area code will be at that time), and we will discuss the possibility of reducing the dosage of some of these. This is simply my way of emphasizing to the patient the fact that you don't *cure* cancer. You can *control* it as long as the defense mechanisms continue to function normally. If a patient goes back to his old eating habits, he will soon be back in trouble again.

Boring Statistics and Exciting Cases

Chapter Twelve

Nothing that has been said so far in this book would be of any significance if there were not some statistics to show that the nutritional approach to the treatment of cancer offers the cancer patient a greater quality and quantity of life than does so-called "orthodox" treatment.

A speaker I recently heard said, "I am not going to bore you with statistics, I am going to do it another way." Well, I am going to bore you with a few statistics, because I feel that they are necessary to prove a point.

Let me repeat something that I said in Chapter Two. Cancer can be divided into two groups. The first group is known as *primary* cancer. This is cancer that is confined to a single area with perhaps a few adjacent lymph nodes involved. The second group is known as *metastatic* cancer. This is *primary* cancer which has spread into other distant areas of the body.

I consider *metastatic* cancer to be almost a different disease than *primary* cancer. I compare the two as I would a flood. The river rises, but the levee protects the low-lying town. Some small low areas may be damaged, but the town, as a whole, survives nicely. Those small areas can be repaired. Suppose, however, that the levee begins to break. Water begins to come into the town. This not only causes more damage, but it also puts more strain on the rest of the levee. This may cause the entire levee to crumble, and now the whole town is destroyed. Thus, while the primary cause of both of the above situations was the flood, whether or not the levee held created two entirely different situations.

Primary cancer is similar to what happens when the levee holds. The damage is small and is restricted to a small area. With proper care, the body can repair it. *Metastatic* cancer is similar to what happens when the levee develops a major leak or breaks entirely. The cancer spreads into distant areas of the body. The damage to the body is infinitely greater, more serious and more difficult to repair. Success or failure in the treatment of *metastatic* cancer depends entirely on how big is the leak, how long it takes to repair, and whether the rest of the levee is strong enough to hold until the leak can be repaired. Thus, while both *primary* and *metastatic* cancer result from the same disease known as "cancer," whether it (the levee) can hold that disease in a small area or whether that defense mechanism (the levee) breaks down and allows the disease to spread widely can create two entirely different situations.

It is for this reason that I separate *primary* cancer and *metastatic* cancer into two different groups.

Statistics are meaningless unless you know how those statistics were derived. In my studies, I went back through my records from 1974 through the end of 1991. All of the patients that I included were diagnosed by physicians other than me and their diagnoses were confirmed by pathology reports. I then compared my results to those of the American Cancer Society. In this section, I want to give the results of my study of patients who had *primary* cancer. I want to stress that in this section I looked at only those patients whose original diagnosis was *primary* cancer, with no metasteses at the time. The results of the patients whose original diagnoses showed metastic disease will be discussed later.

PRIMARY CANCER:

Patients excluded from this study:

It has been my opinion for some years that it may take as long as six months of nutritional therapy for the defense mechanisms of the body to begin to respond. Thus, I excluded from my study all patients with *primary* cancer who died within the first six months of treatment. These were patients whose defense mechanisms had been badly damaged or completely destroyed by their disease, the treatment they had received or a combination of both. Almost all of those in this group who were excluded were patients who had rapidly growing tumors in spite of (or perhaps because of) all of the radiation and/or chemotherapy they had received. They had been told by their radiologist and/or oncologist that their treatments had failed and there was nothing more that could be done. Usually the white blood cells and the body's ability to manufacture white blood cells had been destroyed. The white blood cells are the body's first line of defense against infection and, as mentioned in Chapter Two, are ultimately responsible for destroying cancer cells. Some of the patients had developed severe heart damage, kidney damage, etc. from their treatment. There were, at most, five patients who had a sudden, complete breakdown of their defense mechanisms and within a matter of a few weeks developed large, inoperable tumors. In these cases, no form of treatment was going to be of any value to these patients. Too much damage had already been done to the body. It was possible in some of these patients to improve the quality of their lives, but not the quantity.

Patients included in this study:

I have included in this study of *primary* cancer patients only those patients with whom I have a follow-up of at least two years and who were alive at that time. There were a number of patients left out of this study who were doing well when I last had contact with them, but that contact was for less than two years. I have also included in this study those patients who lived at least six months, but subsequently died.

There are 180 such patients in this study. Thirty different types of cancer are represented. While none of these are the ordinary skin cancers, 10 of them are the deadly malignant melanoma type of skin cancer. From 1974 through 1991, a total of 42 patients have died. Twenty-three of those patients (12.7%) died from causes related to their cancer.

Three of the patients developed metastases while on the program and died. One of them lived 2 years and died at the age of 73. One of them lived 4 years and died at the age of 76. The third one lived 9 years and died at the age of 56. Five other patients developed metastatic disease while on the program but are still alive.

Thirty-nine of the patients on the program did not develop metastases but did die. As mentioned above, 23 died from cancer. Twelve died from causes unrelated to their cancer. Some died from heart attacks and strokes. One died from choking on food; one from a ruptured appendix; and one died in the MGM hotel fire in Las Vegas. Seven died of "cause unknown." These I put in because I had been in contact with these people less than two months prior to their deaths. They were doing well at that time. I was unable to find out the exact cause of their deaths, but it is difficult for me to believe that these people died a cancer death in that short a period of time.

Results:

What all of this means is that out of 180 patients, over a period of 18 years, 87.3% *did not die* from their disease. Even if I concede that the 7 patients who died of "cause unknown" did, indeed, die from cancer, I am still looking at 16.7% of patients who died from their cancer and 83.3% who did not. One hundred and thirty-eight of these patients are still alive. Fifty-eight of these patients (42%) have a follow-up of between two years and four years. Eighty of these patients (58%) have a follow-up of between five and eighteen years. It is important to realize that this is ongoing. By the end of 1992, some new patients would come into the two-year category, and those in the four-year category would move into the five-year category.

I now ask you to compare my results with the statistics of the American Cancer Society for *primary* cancer. The American Cancer Society tells us that in *primary* cancer, with early diagnosis and early treatment with surgery, and/or radiation and/or chemotherapy, eighty-five percent (85%) of the patients *will die* from their disease within five years.

'Nuff said.

METASTATIC CANCER:

Yes, you are going to get more statistics. All of the patients in the study that follows had metastatic cancer when I first saw them. It was not I who made the diagnosis of *metastatic* cancer. These diagnoses were made by other physicians and confirmed by pathology reports.

Patients excluded from this study:

As I stated previously, it is my opinion that it takes as long as six months for the defense mechanisms of the body to respond to nutritional therapy in *primary* cancer patients. In *metastatic* cancer it may take as long as one year. Thus, I have excluded from my study all *metastatic* cancer patients who died within the first year of treatment.[1] The reason for this is the same as stated previously. Most of these patients had developed wide-spread metastases while on radiation and/or chemotherapy and had been told that nothing else could be done. The low white blood cell count and the inability to manufacture white blood cells was there. The heart damage, kidney damage, etc. was there. The total damage to the entire body was greater than in *primary* cancer, and the time needed to repair that damage was longer. Again, it was possible through nutritional therapy to increase the *quality* of life of some of these patients, but not the *quantity*.

Patients included in this study:

I have included in this study of *metastatic* cancer only those patients with whom I have a follow-up of at least two years and who were alive at that time. Again, there were a number of patients left out of this study who were doing well when I last contacted them, but that last contact was for less than two years. I have included in this study all patients who lived at least one year but subsequently died.

There were 108 patients in the study representing 23 different types of cancer. No ordinary skin cancers were included, but 4 of the patients had malignant melanoma with metastases.

1. This is customary protocol. Cancer statistics based on orthodox therapies also eliminate those with incompleted therapy.

Results:

From the period 1974 through 1991 thirty-two of those patients (29.6%) died from their disease. Seven patients developed further metastases while on the program. Three of those seven died from their disease, 3 are still alive and 1 died of a cause unrelated to his disease. A total of 47 patients died. As stated above, 32 died from cancer. Six died of causes unrelated to their disease, and 9 died of cause unknown. Again, "cause unknown" is for the same reason that I used for my *primary* cancer study.

This means that out of 108 patients with *metastatic* cancer, over a period of 18 years, 76 of those patients (70.4%) did not die of their disease. Again, even if I concede that the 9 patients who died of "cause unknown" did, indeed, die from their cancer, I am looking at 37.9% who died from their disease and 62.1% who did not. Sixty-one of those patients are still alive. Thirty of those patients (49%) had a follow-up of between two and four years. Thirty-one of them (51%) had a follow-up of between five and eighteen years. Again, you must realize that this is an ongoing figure, just as I stated for my *primary* cancer patients.

The American Cancer Society tells us that in *metastatic* cancer, with early diagnosis and early treatment with surgery, and/or radiation and/or chemotherapy, only 0.1% (one out of one thousand) of those patients will survive 5 years.

If you consider only those patients who have survived five years or more, this means that my results were 287% better than those reported by the American Cancer Society for the treatment of *metastatic* cancer by "orthodox" methods alone.

CASE HISTORIES

Following are some case histories from my files. The full name is given where permission has been obtained; otherwise, the patient's initials are used.

Case No. 1: Polly Todd

This 59-year-old woman was seen by me for the first time on 1/10/75 with the history that she had her left breast removed one month previously because of carcinoma. Three positive nodes had been found. I will let the patient tell you the rest of her history in her own words:

"It was recommended by a prominent physician that I be a part of an experiment in a (then) new chemotherapy program. For a second opinion I went to another city where I had a personal contact with the head of a large hospital. There they told me that my odds of survival were slim, and that I should be treated with strong doses of chemotherapy and radiation. At this point, a friend told me about the Laetrile-nutritional program, which I chose."

The lady was placed on a nutritional program at that time and she has remained on it ever since. She is now 79 years old, in good health, and she has had no recurrence of her disease.

In a recent letter the patient said, "None of the above people on the chemotherapy program lived beyond 1 1/2 years. Friends who scoffed at our choice then have much more respect now because others choosing the conventional treatment are gone, while I survive!"

Case No. 2: Sue Tarbutton

This 50 year-old woman was seen by me for the first time on 10/26/83 with a history that one week before she had a lump removed from her right breast which was found to be malignant. She did not want to have a mastectomy and wanted to go on a nutritional program.

114

She has now been on the program for ten years, has had no recurrence of her disease and is quite well.

Case No. 3: Elizabeth Winschel

This 51-year-old woman was first seen by me on 10/11/76. Four months before she had been found to have carcinoma of the colon with malignant cells in the abdominal fluid. She had four chemotherapy treatments but discontinued them because they made her so ill. She was started on a nutritional program. Now, seventeen years later, she continues to do well with no recurrence at the primary site of her disease and no metastases.

Case No. 4: Wasley Krogdahl

This 60-year-old man was first seen by me on 4/20/79. In November, 1977, he had been diagnosed with having carcinoma of the urinary bladder. The tumor was removed. In February, 1979, three more tumors were removed. He was started on a nutritional program. In April, 1981, and again in November, 1982, some small tumors were removed from his bladder.

He and his wife came to visit me just recently. He is now 75 years old. He has had no further recurrence of his disease. He looks well, says he is feeling well and his wife says, "He is just as hard-headed as ever."

Case No. 5: Beverly Batson

This 70-year-old woman was seen by me for the first time on 9/19/88. She had one-half of her stomach removed one month prior because of carcinoma. She received no radiation or chemotherapy. She has been on her nutritional program for five years. Now at the age of 75, she remains well with no recurrence at the primary site or with any metastases.

Case No. 6: Jean Henshall

This 48-year-old woman, that I saw for the first time on 9/8/87, had a history of being diagnosed ten months previously with malignant myeloma (a cancer which affects the bone). Her disease affected the bones in the pelvic area. She had received some radiation to that area which relieved the pain. She was started on a nutritional program which pretty much followed the protocol outlined in Chapter Eleven. However, after she had been off of her Laetrile injections for a few months, she was aware that she did not feel as well as she did while on them. She went back on some injections for a few months, and she felt much better. The injections were again stopped, and she remained on the Laetrile pills. This time she noticed no difference. She has now been on the program for six years and is doing well. "I'm doing everything. Even housework is a joy to me because I *can* do it."

Case No. 7: R.H.

This 43-year-old woman was seen by me for the first time on 10/26/79. Two months prior she had been found to have carcinoma of the ovary with metastases throughout the abdomen. She was, at that time, on chemotherapy. We discussed nutritional therapy—what it would do and what it would not do. I saw her next on 11/13/79. She had two chemotherapy treatments by this time, but she had decided to discontinue them and go on a nutritional program.

She stayed on the program until 1982, decided that she was "cured" at that time and went off of the program completely. I saw her on 6/19/84. At this time, she had a tumor running from her right pelvis up into the right upper quadrant of her abdomen. She went back on her nutritional program. I saw her again on 8/1/84. She was feeling very well. The edges of the tumor were much softer and much more difficult to define. When I saw her on 9/2/84, the edges of the tumor were even softer than before.

I did not see her again until 8/20/85. She had been off of her program for 7 or 8 months. Why? It's a long story, and because of "privileged information" I am not free to discuss it. The tumor had enlarged and was now causing abdominal pain and some swelling in the right leg. I put her back on her program, which included some Laetrile injections, and recommended that she have the tumor surgically removed. On 10/1/85, the patient called me to say that she had undergone surgery. She said that the surgeon had found 5 well walled-off tumors that were easily removed. The pathology report, she said, showed mostly "dead" cancer cells.

In 1988 the patient went off her nutritional program. In 1991 she developed a bowel obstruction from her cancer and now has a colostomy. She did go back on her program again and has remained on it. In the three years that have passed since that time, there has been no recurrence of her disease.

Case No. 8: Joan Dewiel

This 45-year-old woman first was seen by me on 1/28/80 with a history of having been found to have carcinoma of the colon in September, 1979. Surgery was done, there were no metastases, and she received no radiation or chemotherapy. She was placed on a nutritional program. That was 14 years ago. She is now 59 years old and has had no recurrence of her disease.

Case No. 9: Rex Perry

This 42-year-old man that I first saw on 6/27/79 with a history of having malignant lymphoma, which was originally diagnosed in August, 1978. He had 8 months of chemotherapy, which he tolerated very well. His doctors felt, however, that there was a significant amount of disease still present. They wanted to do several more months of chemotherapy and follow this with total body radiation. The patient did not want to do this because of his concern about what it would do to his immune system. He chose, instead, to use the nutritional approach.

It has now been almost 15 years since he started his nutritional therapy. The most satisfying part of such a case history is that this patient has had no further problem with his disease. He is well and very active.

Case No. 10: Pauline Wilcox

This 58-year-old woman was seen by me for the first time on 6/14/85 with a history of having had her left breast removed because of carcinoma in 1983. She received no radiation or chemotherapy.

She was placed on a nutritional program at that time. Since she had already gone for two years without any problem, I used only the Laetrile tablets as that part of her nutritional program. She did well on that program until 1988, when she went off of her diet and was taking her vitamins, enzymes and Laetrile only now and then. In November, 1988, she developed a small lesion on her chest wall. This was removed and found to be a spread of her cancer. She went back on her nutritional program again, except this time I added a series of intravenous Laetrile injections. Since then she has had two other small lesions removed from her chest wall which contained some cancer cells. Most importantly, chest x-rays and bone scans done on both occasions were normal. She remains in good health today. As this patient said to me recently, "My doctor is amazed."

BORING STATISTICS AND EXCITING CASES

Case No. 11: Connie Stork

This 24-year-old woman first was seen by me on 2/26/75. Her history was that in 1970 she had been found to have a malignant tumor of the brain. The tumor was partially removed. This was followed by 25 radiation treatments. In October, 1974, another large mass of tumor was removed, but much of the tumor remained. She was told that she had all of the radiation she could have. She was started on a nutritional program.

Now, some 19 years later, Connie has had no recurrence of her tumor. She did have greatly impaired vision as the result of her tumors in 1970 and 1974, and this has progressed to blindness. However, she is still very much alive and is blessed with a healthy mind and healthy body.

Case No. 12: Irene Dirks

This 59-year-old woman was seen for the first time on 8/19/80. Her history was that six weeks before I saw her she had been found to have a very low hemoglobin (anemia). She was given blood. Her workup showed that she had a gastric ulcer, but it was questionable whether she had any bleeding from that ulcer. I discussed with her at that time a nutritional program that included some changes in her diet, some vitamins and a small amount of Laetrile by mouth. These changes were obviously not sufficient, because in March, 1981, she began having occasional vaginal bleeding. Two months later this bleeding was found to come from endometrial carcinoma (cancer of the lining of the uterus). A hysterectomy was done, and she was put on the full nutritional program. Now, some 14 years later, she has had no recurrence of her disease and at the age of 73 is quite well and very active.

Case No. 13: Doris Dickson

This 50-year-old woman was first seen on 5/14/85 with a history of having had a node removed from the left side of her neck in 1979. From this a diagnosis of lymphatic leukemia was made. She had one chemotherapy treatment, but this made her so ill she discontinued it. She went on a nutritional program of her own which she stayed on until six months prior to the time I first saw her. She stated that for the past two or three months she had not felt well and that a recent blood count showed a 21,000 white cell count. A white cell count done on the day I saw her was 24,000. (A normal count is about 5,000 to 10,500.)

Mrs. Dickson was started on my nutritional program. I did not feel in her case that the intravenous Laetrile was necessary, so I used just the Laetrile tablets as that part of her program. One month later Mrs. Dickson reported that she was feeling much better. Her white cell count was down to 17,300. Her white cell count continued to drop and by November, 1985, it was down to 9,700.

In June, 1991, Mrs. Dickson reported a gradual increase in fatigue. Her white-cell count was 13,700. I reviewed her nutritional program and found some slips here-and-there that needed to be corrected. By October of that year her cell count was down to 10,700. In a recent letter from her, Mrs. Dickson reports that she is doing well.

Case No. 14: T.P.

This 59-year-old man that was seen for the first time on 7/18/80. His history was that one month prior to this a routine x-ray showed a mass in his right lung. A biopsy showed this to be carcinoma. Five radiation treatments were given followed by one chemotherapy treatment that made him so ill he discontinued that whole program. He was started on my nutritional program.

120

An x-ray done in January, 1981, showed that the tumor in his right lung was completely gone. Let me quote from a letter I received from him on January 23, 1981:

"They were surprised here at [hospital name omitted] comparing the x-ray of last June and the one I just received.... Hope you understand what I am trying to say. I was really tickled when I learned the tumor was gone, and I thought of you right away. I know in my heart it was the Amygdalin and will never think differently.

"The doctor I had at the hospital in June said it was probably the 5 radiation treatments I had. They just don't want to admit [it was the Amygdalin], I guess."

My last contact with this patient was in April, 1993. At that time he was doing very well.

Case No. 15: Helyne Victor

This 54-year-old woman was first seen on 6/7/74. In 1967 she had her right breast removed because of cancer. In 1970 she had her left breast removed, also because of cancer. She had received no radiation or chemotherapy after either surgery. While yearly check-ups had failed to find any spread of her disease, this woman just didn't feel well and wanted to get on a good nutritional program.

Mrs. Victor tells her story best. This is from a letter she wrote to the Ohio State Medical Board on April 5. 1975:

"My health has not been good and it was approximately a year ago that I found myself going downhill as far as my health was concerned, not knowing what to do or to whom to go for help. My husband and I began to read and research various avenues for nutritional help or aid.

"I felt very strongly that my poor health may have been due partly to faulty nutrition. After reading materials on proper diets, etc., I heard of Dr. Binzel and had heard that he did treat patients with a nutritional program. So, I called him and made an appointment....

"Following a good diet, as he suggested, and taking multiple vitamins for the past year, I can honestly say that I feel like a different person. My health has improved 100%, and I'm feeling like my old self and extremely happy with the results...."

Mrs. Victor continues to do well. She is now 74 years old and in a recent letter she said of herself and her husband, "We enjoy life and travel a lot."

Case No. 16: M.S.

This 62-year-old woman was first seen on 12/6/78. One month previously she had a mole removed from her back. This mole turned out to be a malignant melanoma. She had no radiation or chemotherapy.

She was placed on a nutritional program. She is now 77 years old, quite well and quite active. She has had small a skin cancer removed from her face, but this was not melanoma and was unrelated to her previous disease.

I bring this case to your attention because melanoma is a highly malignant disease which frequently metastasizes rapidly to the liver. This woman was one of 10 patients that I saw with primary malignant melanoma (it had not spread to any other area). To the best of my knowledge, none of those patients have developed metastatic disease.

Case No. 17: B.D.

This 62-year-old woman was seen by me for the first time on 5/22/84. In January, 1980, she had been found to have malignant lymphoma. She received chemotherapy from January, 1980, through November, 1980. In March, 1982, she developed a small nodule in the back portion of her left neck area and a few months later a larger nodule in the right mandibular angle (jaw). She placed herself on a pretty good nutritional program at that time and the nodules had not progressed at all in size.

I up-graded the nutritional program of this patient by adding Vitamin A and Laetrile to what she was already doing. She was followed closely by her family doctor for the next two years. He could not detect any enlargements of these nodules. I saw her again on 4/30/86. I felt that the nodule in the right mandibular angle was the same size as before but was firmer and more movable. I thought the nodule on the left side of the neck was the same size but much firmer than before. The next time I saw this patient was on 2/18/91. I could not find any nodules at all.

It has now been 10 years since she started on her nutritional program. In a recent letter she said, "I am doing well and leading an active life...I continue to take all of the vitamins that you prescribed and I never miss a dose."

Case No. 18: B.W.

This 44-year-old woman was seen for the first time on 2/6/81. She had been found one month prior to have carcinoma of the descending colon with 7 positive lymph nodes. A colostomy was not required. She received no radiation or chemotherapy.

She was started on a nutritional program. Now, some 13 years later, she has had no recurrence of her disease and leads a normal, active life.

What is so unusual about this patient? She had cancer of the colon with metastases. The odds of her surviving 5 years were one in one-thousand. Yet, she lives a normal life with no recurrence of her disease after 13 years.

Case No. 19: Alice Silverthorn

This 46-year-old woman was seen by me for the first time on 1/5/76. Her left breast had been removed in 1971 because of carcinoma. This was followed by radiation and chemotherapy. She had just been told that her disease had now spread to the cervical vertebrae (neck), her left rib cage and the vertebrae in her lower back. Her doctors wanted to give her more chemotherapy, but she did not want it. She wanted to go on a nutritional program.

When she started her nutritional program, she was having much pain. Within a month, the pain began to subside. In April, 1976, she began having more pain in her rib cage and in her lower back. She was put back on her intravenous Laetrile three times weekly for two weeks. The pain again subsided. In August of that year she began to have some pain once more in her rib cage. She was given intravenous Laetrile twice weekly for three weeks. Again the pain subsided. It has now been 18 years since she first started on her program. She is 64 years old and doing very well.

Let me share with you part of a letter I recently received from Mrs. Silverthorn:

"I remember only too well the fear and desperation, yes, and downright helplessness, I felt when the doctors at (hospital name deleted) told me the cancer had metastasized to my bones. It was a sentence of 'death.' I was told I would need to start chemo-treatments immediately. There was even talk of taking the pituitary gland out at some later date. I had already had a radical left breast operation and was treated with mustard gas, cobalt and male hormones. I had enough of torture! ! !

"When a friend told me about your nutritional approach to treating diseases, I was ready to try it. Even though we both knew my chances of survival were slim, together, we were willing to take on the challenge of fighting for my life. Now, thank God, you can claim me as one of your survivors.

BORING STATISTICS AND EXCITING CASES

"I hope you include in your book how we feel, and just how difficult it is for those of us who were supposed to die, when the medical profession and well-meaning, intelligent people make the suggestion that the only reason we are alive is because it was a mis-diagnosis or the disease has gone into a 'spontaneous' remission. Most people make us feel like psychiatric patients. It is difficult to explain miracles, yet, that is what happened."

Case No. 20: Grace Laman

This 59-year-old woman was seen for the first time on 10/5/76. She had been diagnosed as having carcinoma of the pancreas six months prior to this. The only thing that had been done surgically was to run a tube from her bile duct to the outside. She was on chemotherapy for two months but stopped it herself because it made her so ill. She was told at that time that she had only 6 months to live. She was placed on a nutritional program.

Let me quote part of a letter I received from her almost two years later (9/23/78):

"I was [recently] put through a new scanner which showed that my tumor had reduced to the size of a tennis ball. It had been the size of [the doctor's] hand, so he said."

Now, 18 years later, she is 77 years old. In the letter which accompanied her picture she said, "This is my activity picture of me *eating out,* which I do very well."

Note: With surgery and/or radiation and/or chemotherapy the chances of surviving more than one year with cancer of the pancreas are about 1 in 10,000.

Case No. 21: E.D.

This 57-year-old man was first seen on 4/28/92 (and for that reason is not included in my statistical study) with a history of a diagnosis of carcinoma of the left lung 10 months previously. Surgery had been done followed by one chemotherapy treatment. This made him so ill that he discontinued it. He was then given 25 radiation treatments ending in December, 1991. In March, 1992, x-rays showed extensive growth of the tumors in that lung. He was placed on a nutritional program.

X-rays done in July, 1993, showed no further growth of the tumors in the left lung. X-rays done in November, 1993, showed that the tumors had all become scar tissue. In the most recen letter I received from him he stated that he was feeling so well that "I have no right to complain, so I have to cuss a lot about taxes, politicians, etc."

These statistics and case histories have focused primarily upon the extension of the patient's life span. That's certainly important, but the *quality* of life is also important. We will deal with that issue next.

PATIENT SURVIVAL (5-yrs or more)

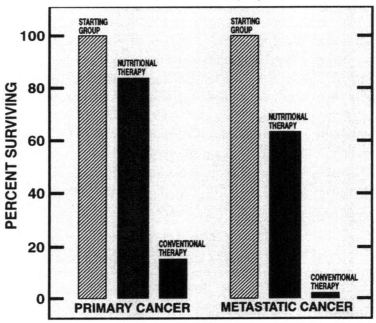

The Quality of Life

Chapter Thirteen

In the previous chapter I talked mostly about the quantity of life (the length of life) that I was able to obtain in the cancer patient through nutritional therapy. Now I want to talk about quality of life. The next few patients that I am going to discuss have all died. However, even though they died, they were able, with the help of nutritional therapy, to have a much finer quality of life than could have been reasonably expected.

The first case I want to discuss is that of a patient I will call "Mr. R.H." I saw this 73-year-old man for the first time in November, 1981. Seven months prior to this he had been found to have cancer of the prostate. He received 35 radiation treatments. A scan done before the radiation showed no tumor activity in any of the bones. A scan done a few months after the radiation did show tumor activity in some of the bones. It was at this point that he decided to go on nutritional therapy.

In August, 1982, he began to have some pain in his left hip. Several doctors told him that they were sure that this was from the spread of his cancer and wanted to do more radiation. I suggested that he see an orthopedic surgeon and say nothing about his prostate cancer. The orthopedic surgeon found that he had a ligament strain, put him on some exercises and in a few weeks the pain was gone. In 1985 he developed some heart problems, but these were easily controlled by medication.

Mr. R.H. died in December, 1993, at the age of 85. My last contact with him was in October, 1991. At that time he was well, traveling a lot and enjoying life. So here was a man who had cancer of the prostate with metastases who not only lived 12 years, but also had at least 10 good-quality years. The American Cancer Society says the possibility of surviving five years with metastatic cancer is only about 1 out of 1,000.

The next is the story about a woman I will call "Mrs. H.R." She was 68 years old when I first saw her in July, 1977. Her history was that in 1974 she had her right breast removed because of cancer. Some radiation was done and was followed by 2 years of chemotherapy. Following the chemotherapy, her left breast was removed for "precautionary reasons." She was now beginning to develop metastatic skin lesions and wanted to go on nutritional therapy. This woman didn't feel well. She had very little energy to do anything.

Within one month she was beginning to feel better, and two months later she called me to say that she was feeling "very well." Over the next 9 years she did have some more nodules develop on the skin in the breast area. A few of them became uncomfortable and she had them surgically removed. The important thing was, that during all of this time, she felt well and lived a normal life. She lived with her son and his family. Her family was from a foreign country. Every summer during those nine years she was able to go and to spend at least two months with her family.

THE QUALITY OF LIFE

Sometime in 1986, someone talked her into having some radiation done on her chest wall. She never really recovered from that, went gradually downhill and died in January, 1987, at the age of 77. Shortly after that I received the following note from her son:

"I regret to inform you that my mother died on January 18, of lung and heart failure. Her lungs were completely invaded with cancer. I am convinced that the radiation therapy she had a year ago was the cause of her demise. In any case, I wish to thank you for giving her 10 years of dignified, healthy life that she would otherwise not have had."

The third case I want to talk about is that of "Mr. R.C." I first saw this 65-year-old man in November, 1976. Two months prior to this he had been found to have cancer of the prostate which had already metastasized to his right ribs. A transurethral resection had been done on the prostate gland. Neither radiation nor chemotherapy had been recommended because, he was told, the disease had already spread too far. He was put on a nutritional program.

This man was a "worrier." Every little ache or pain he got made him sure it was his cancer. It took a lot of support over several years to get him to realize that there were a number of things, other than cancer, which could cause these aches and pains. It wasn't until May, 1979, that I finally got him convinced. At that time he was having some low back pain. He was sure that this was from the spread of his cancer. He saw a good orthopedic surgeon, who did all of the tests, and found that this pain was from an old back problem (a degenerative disc). With some limitation of activity and some exercises, within one month the pain was gone. It was not until 11 years later, at the age of 76, that he began to get into serious trouble. In

June, 1987, he began having a lot of pain. A bone scan at that time showed many "hot" areas. He had 10 radiation treatments in August, 1987, which relieved much of the pain but left him very weak. He died 5 months later.

Here, again, was a man with metastatic cancer. He was essentially told that there was nothing that could be done. Yes, he did die from his disease, but, in the meantime, he got 11 years of quality living.

"Mrs. A.B." was an 83-year-old woman when I first saw her in 1987. Just a few weeks earlier, she had a nodule removed from a breast which was found to be malignant. She was also found at this time to have chronic lymphatic leukemia. She did not want any radiation or chemotherapy, and I am not sure that her doctors, because of her age, were enthusiastic about using those forms of treatment.

She was placed on a nutritional program. She did very well. She had many interests and was able to pursue these with her usual vigor. She died 6 years later at the age of 89, but felt well and was active during most of that time. It is difficult to say whether she lived any longer because of her nutritional program, but there is no doubt that the quality of her life was far better than would have been expected had she done nothing at all.

"Mr. N.D." was 74 years old when I first saw him in August, 1979. One month prior to this he had been found to have cancer of the lower colon. He refused surgery because this would have necessitated a colostomy. He dreaded that idea.

He was put on a nutritional program. He did continue to have some rectal bleeding from time-to-time, but this was never a problem as far as causing anemia. He died 7 years later at the age of 81 from a heart attack.

Here, again, it is the *quality* of life that is so important. In this man's opinion a colostomy was a terrible thing to have. If he had a colostomy, whatever years of life he had left would have been ruined. As it was, he was able to live out the rest of his natural life with physical comfort and peace of mind.

God grant that all of us may do the same!

Treat the Cause,
Not the Symptom!

Chapter Fourteen

The most logical question for anyone to ask at this point is, "If nutritional therapy is as successful as you say, why isn't every doctor in this county using it?" The only accurate answer would be, of course, to ask every doctor in this country. Thus, the answers I give to this question are my opinion.

Is there politics involved with cancer therapy? I have every reason to believe that there is. It is not the purpose of this book to get into the political aspects of cancer therapy. For those who would like to pursue that subject in-depth, I would suggest that you read *World Without Cancer* by G. Edward Griffin. Mr. Griffin has also produced an excellent audio tape on the subject entitled *The Politics of Cancer Therapy.* [1]

Is money a factor? For some doctors it may be. There is a lot of money to be made in surgery, radiation and chemotherapy. From twenty years of experience, I know that simply putting a patient on a good diet, giving them

1. These items can be obtained from American Media, PO Box 4646, Westlake Village, CA 91359, or call (800) 282-2873.

some vitamins, enzymes, etc. and checking on them from time-to-time does not produce much revenue.

More importantly, I am convinced that most doctors in this country are dedicated individuals. They will do anything that they think will help their patients. However, the problem with most of the doctors is that they are "tumor-oriented." They have been trained to be "lump and bump" doctors with no concept of how nutrition relates to disease.

Here's what I mean. When a patient is found to have a tumor, the only thing the doctor discusses with that patient is what he intends to do about the tumor. If a patient with a tumor is receiving radiation or chemotherapy, the only question that is asked is, "How is the tumor doing?" No one ever asks how the patient is doing. In my medical training, I remember well seeing patients who were getting radiation and/or chemotherapy. The tumor would get smaller and smaller, but the patient would be getting sicker and sicker. At autopsy we would hear, "Isn't that marvelous! The tumor is gone!" Yes, it was, but so was the patient. How many millions of times are we going to have to repeat these scenarios before we realize that we are treating the wrong thing?

In *primary* cancer, with only a few exceptions, the tumor is neither health-endangering nor life-threatening. I am going to repeat that statement. In *primary* cancer, with few exceptions, the tumor is neither health-endangering nor life-threatening. What *is* health-endangering and life-threatening is the *spread* of that disease through the rest of the body.

There is nothing in surgery that will prevent the spread of cancer. There is nothing in radiation that will prevent the spread of the disease. There is nothing in chemotherapy that will prevent the spread of the disease. How do we

TREAT THE CAUSE, NOT THE SYMPTOM!

know? Just look at the statistics! There is a statistic known as "survival time." Survival time is defined as that interval of time between when the diagnosis of cancer is first made in a given patient and when that patient dies from his disease. In the past fifty years, tremendous progress has been made in the early diagnosis of cancer. In that period of time, tremendous progress had been made in the surgical ability to remove tumors. Tremendous progress has been made in the use of radiation and chemotherapy in their ability to shrink or destroy tumors. But, *the survival time of the cancer patient today is no greater than it was fifty years ago.* What does this mean? It obviously means that *we are treating the wrong thing!* We are treating the symptom - the tumor, and we are doing absolutely nothing to prevent the spread of the disease. *The only thing known to mankind today that will prevent the spread of cancer within the body is for that body's own defense mechanisms to once again function normally.* That's what nutritional therapy does. It treats the defense mechanism, not the tumor.

The woman with a lump in her breast is not going to die from that lump. The man with a nodule in his prostate gland is not going to die from that nodule. What may kill both of those people is the spread of that disease through the rest of their bodies. They got their disease because of a breakdown of their defense mechanisms. The only thing that is going to prevent the spread of their disease is to correct the problem in those defense mechanisms. Doesn't it seem logical then, that we should be a lot less concerned with "What are we going to do about the tumor?" and a lot more concerned about what we are going to do about their defense mechanisms?

135

ALIVE AND WELL

Please note the statement that I made previously: Nutritional therapy treats the defense mechanism, not the tumor. I do not want anyone reading this book to think, "If I get cancer, I'll go on a nutritional program, and my tumor will magically disappear." No, it won't. Once a tumor has become firmly established in the body, the body accepts that tumor as normal tissue and will not attack it. No tumor is ever more than ten percent "cancer" cells. By "cancer" cells I mean the highly malignant, undifferentiated cells. The other ninety percent of that tumor is made up of, what I choose to call, "transitional" cells. These are cells which, while they show the effects of cancer, retain enough of their own characteristics to allow their origin to be identified. That is, you can tell whether these cells are breast tissue, liver tissue, or whatever. For reasons not fully understood at this time, the body will not attack those "transitional" cells. The body may kill off the undifferentiated cells, but these will be replaced with scar tissue. This is what happened to the patients in Case Histories #20 and #21. The body will not attack the "transitional" cells. Thus, the tumor remains. The body attempts to wall-off the tumor with a fibrous sack. This is what happened to the patient in Case History #7.

I am sure that there are still some of you who are concerned about "What are you going to do about the tumor?" There are only three times when I am concerned about the tumor:

1. If the tumor, because of its size or position, is interfering with some vital function, you have to deal with the tumor by whatever means are best available.

2. If the tumor, because of its size or position, is causing pain, you have to deal with the tumor by whatever means are available.

TREAT THE CAUSE, NOT THE SYMPTOM!

3. If the presence of the tumor presents a psychological problem for the patient, have it removed.

In general, if the tumor is easily accessible and if the patient wishes to do so, I like to have the tumor removed. Not all doctors doing nutritional therapy agree with that. I feel that by removing the tumor the body has one less thing with which to cope. If the tumor is remote, not causing any problem and the patient agrees, I leave the tumor alone. Again, I stress the fact that the tumor is merely a symptom, not a cause. If you take care of the body, the body will take care of the tumor. That doesn't mean that the tumor will go away, but it is unlikely to cause a problem.

I am not opposed to the use of radiation. I am not opposed to the use of chemotherapy. There are times when a small amount of radiation for a short period of time can relieve pain and/or be life-saving to a patient. There are times when a small amount of chemotherapy for a short period of time can do the same. It is not the use of these that I so vehemently oppose, it is their abuse. The theory used in this country is that, if a little does some good, a whole lot more will do a whole lot better. Patients are getting radiation and chemotherapy who do not need it. Those who do need it are often getting far more than they need, thereby doing them much more harm than good.

The ultimate question is, "Does nutritional therapy work?" That depends on how you define "work." If you are tumor oriented and are looking for something to make the tumor magically disappear, no, it doesn't. If you are looking for something that will prevent the disease from spreading and save the life of the patient, yes, it does.

I have not said anything about the cost of nutritional therapy. I have no way of knowing what other doctors charge for their services. I do know the cost to the patient for their vitamins, enzymes, and Laetrile. I do know that for my patients their total cost for one *year,* including my services, is about one-half the cost of *one* radiation treatment and about one-third the cost of *one* chemotherapy treatment.

Is there any hope that nutritional therapy will ever be accepted by the medical profession? In my opinion, it is not a matter of "if," it is only a matter of "when." As a patient of mine said to me several years ago, "If doctors in this country don't start going to nutrition, the patients are going to stop going to the doctors." The use of nutrition in the prevention and treatment of disease will come from the ground up, not from the top down. People are getting more nutritionally oriented and are going to insist that their doctors do the same.

In regard to the treatment of cancer with nutritional therapy, before this comes about, two things are going to have to happen:

> 1. The medical profession is going to have to realize that they have been treating the wrong thing. They are going to have to realize that, as long as they continue to treat just the tumor alone, they are going to continue to get the same poor results that they have always had.

> 2. The medical profession is going to have to accept the fact that the quality and quantity of life for the cancer patient obtained through nutritional therapy is far superior to anything available through our present modalities. In simpler terms, these people on nutritional therapy feel better and live longer.

I, most certainly, do not want to leave the impression that everything about nutrition that can be known is now known. The very opposite is true. We have only just begun to scratch the surface of our understanding of the relationship between nutrition and disease. It is my opinion that we must first understand the defense mechanisms of the body. Why do these defense mechanisms respond so rapidly is some situations and so slowly in others? What systems of the body are involved in the defense mechanisms? In what order do they respond? Once we have the answer to these questions we can then determine what nutritional ingredients are necessary to keep those systems of the body functioning normally.

The fact that we do not have the answers to the above-stated questions does not mean, however, that we should not use the information that we do have to its fullest extent. The pure medical scientist will not use any form of treatment until he fully understands why it works and how it works. The good practitioner, on the other hand, will use any form of treatment that works, even if he does not understand exactly why and how it works.

There are many examples of good practitioners in the annals of medical history. Dr. Semmelweis, in 1860, insisted that all doctors wash their hands before delivering a baby because, by so doing, it eliminated "child bed fever." He knew it worked, but he did not know why or how it worked. He was removed from the hospital staff and ostracized by the medical community. It was not until about the time that Dr. Semmelweis died in 1865 that Dr. Lister discovered bacteria. Dr. Lister was able to prove that Dr. Semmelweis was right and why he was right. I doubt that Dr. Fleming in 1925 knew why he could cure pneumonia by giving his patients moldy bread. He knew it worked, but he did not know why or how it worked. It wasn't until some time later that he discovered a fungus in moldy bread that could kill certain bacteria. This fungus eventually became known as penicillin. Dr. Fleming was ridiculed by the medical profession for his work. It would be another fifteen years before penicillin came into use. By then, thousands of patients had died from pneumonia.

ALIVE AND WELL

So it is with nutritional therapy in the treatment of cancer. I hope in this book that I have been able to present sufficient evidence to show that it works, even though at this time we do not know exactly why and how it works.

After all is said and done, the true measurement of a good physician is not necessarily how much he knows. It is, instead, how willing he is to search for, find and then *use* whatever forms of treatment, which in his opinion, will give his patients the very best chance to remain...

ALIVE AND WELL.

INDEX

American Cancer Society: 108,
111, 113, 128
Amygdalin (See Laetrile)
Anderson, Professor: 67 - 70,
72 - 73, 76

Bath, John: 81, 89
Batson, Beverly: 60, 115
Benzaldehyde: 23, 47 - 48
Beta-glucosidase: 23, 47
Binzel, Betty: 13 - 15, 18, 20,
29, 35, 39, 52, 75, 77 - 80, 95
Binzel, Bill: 53 - 55, 87 - 89
Binzel, Michelle: 53 - 56
Binzel, Rick: 53 - 56
Bohanon, Judge Luther: 13, 15,
17 - 18, 40 - 45, 86
Bradford, Robert: 13 - 14, 18, 34
Bromalin: 98
Burk, Dr. Dean: 21 - 26, 97, 101

Califano, Joseph A.: 40, 43
Cancer: Throughout
Cancer, metastatic: 16, 30 - 31,
51, 107 - 114, 128, 130
Cancer, primary: 16, 30 - 31,
107 - 114, 134
Carcinoma: 60, 114 - 121, 123,
125
Case histories: Throughout, with
specific cases on 114 - 126
Chemotherapy: See orthodox
treatment
Chymotrypsin: 22 - 25, 98,
101 - 103
Coe, Ken: 14 - 18
Coe, Ruthie: 5, 13 - 14, 35, 76,
86
Coffman, Judge Evelyn: 66, 68,
89 - 96

Committee for Freedom of
Choice in Cancer Therapy:
13, 21, 27, 29, 34
Contreras, Dr. Ernesto: 21 - 26,
97, 101
Cyanide: 23, 42, 47 - 49, 54

Dewiel, Joan: 117
Dickson, Doris: 120
Diet: Throughout
Dirks, Irene: 62 - 63, 119

Enzymes: 22 - 26, 28, 47, 54,
98 - 99, 101 - 103, 106, 118,
134, 137

Food and Drug Administration
(FDA): 8, 13, 15 - 19,
39 - 45, 47 - 49, 53, 55, 64,
86 - 87

Glucose: 23, 47
Griffin, G. Edward: 5, 8, 11, 12,
19 - 20, 40, 48, 108, 133
Griffin, Patricia: 34

Haines, Joe: 95 - 96
Halstead, Dr. Bruce: 13 - 14,
16 - 18
Henshall, Jean: 61, 116
Hodgkins Disease: 67 - 68, 85
Hofbauer, Joey: 67 - 71, 73, 76
Hofbauer, John: 68 - 69
Hydrogen cyanide (HCN)
See cyaninde

John Birch Society: 20, 27

Kell, George: 34 - 36
Kennedy, Donald: 40, 43, 45

141

INDEX

Krebs, Jr., Dr. Ernst T.: 5, 21 - 26, 29 - 30, 97, 101
Krogdahl, Wasley: 60, 115

Laetrile: Throughout
Laman, Grace: 125 - 126

Macalester College: 53 - 54
Magnesium: 26
Manganese: 26
Manner, Dr. Harold: 54 - 55
McDonald, Dr. Lawrence P.: 27, 55
Megazyme Forte: 98
Melanoma: 110, 112, 122
Michaelis, Steve: 20 - 21, 27
Myeloma: 61, 116

National Cancer Institute (NCI): 52 - 53
Navarro, Dr. Manuel: 21 - 26, 97, 101
Nieper, Dr. Hans: 21 - 26, 97, 101
Nitrilosides: 21, 23 - 25, 98, 100 - 101
Nutritional therapy: Throughout

Ohio, State Medical Board: 8, 34 - 37, 57, 62 - 72, 80, 85 - 96, 121
Orthodox Treatment (Radiation, chemotherapy, surgery): Throughout

Pangamic Acid: 98

Perry, Rex: 62, 117 - 118
Pro-A-Mulsion: 98

Radiation: See orthodox treatment
Richardson, Dr. John: 34
Rutherford, Glen L.: 39 - 40, 42

Sakai, Dr. Shigeaki: 21 - 26, 97, 101
Schachter, Dr. Michael: 72 - 74, 76
Silverthorn, Alice: 64 - 65, 124 - 125
Sloan-Kettering: 51
St. Louis University School of Medicine: 19
Stork, Connie: 62 - 63, 119
Sugiura, Dr. Kanematsu: 51 - 52

Tarbutton, Sue: 59, 114 - 115
Thiocyanate: 48, 100
Todd, Polly: 58, 114
Trypsin: 22 - 25, 98, 101 - 103

Victor, Helyne: 65, 121
Vitamin A: 26, 54, 100
Vitamin B: 26, 48
Vitamin B$_{12}$: 26, 48
Vitamin C: 25 - 26, 98, 100
Vitamin E: 98

Wilcox, Pauline: 61, 118
Winschel, Elizabeth: 59, 115

Zinc: 26, 98 - 99